Dr Sonica Krish

Ayurveda professio
columnist, editor a
author of *Herbal H*
received a wide response.

She may be contacted at sonicakrishan@gmail.com, http://drsonicakrishan.blogspot.in/, www.drsonicakrishan.com and http://www.herboveda.co.in/.

Home Remedies

to prevent and
cure common ailments

Sonica Krishan

RUPA

Published by
Rupa Publications India Pvt. Ltd 2007
7/16, Ansari Road, Daryaganj
New Delhi 110002

Sales centres:
Allahabad Bengaluru Chennai
Hyderabad Jaipur Kathmandu
Kolkata Mumbai

Copyright © Sonica Krishan 2007

All rights reserved.
No part of this publication may be reproduced, transmitted,
or stored in a retrieval system, in any form or by any means,
electronic, mechanical, photocopying, recording or otherwise,
without the prior permission of the publisher.

ISBN: 978-81-291-1190-6

Second impression 2013

10 9 8 7 6 5 4 3 2

The moral right of the author has been asserted.

Typeset by Prints of Desire, Okhla Industrial Area, New Delhi

Printed at Saurabh Printers, Noida

This book is sold subject to the condition that it shall not, by way
of trade or otherwise, be lent, resold, hired out, or otherwise circulated,
without the publisher's prior consent, in any form of binding or cover
other than that in which it is published.

ACKNOWLEDGEMENTS

My sincere thanks and gratitude:

- To the Almighty who has blessed me with the faith and trust to reach to the world and propagate the natural ways of healing.
- To my publishers Rupa and co. who have been great support and guide in my enterprise.
- To my husband, CA Alok Krishan, who has been highly encouraging and motivating.
- To my parents and my mother-in-law for their moral assistance.
- To my children, Ishita and Ishan, who are true examples of endurance and love for me.
- And to the readers who exhibit keen interest and acceptance in publications and books that are in harmony with the natural therapies.
- Please send feedback / comments at drsonica@rediffmail.com. They are a source of motivation.

THE RIGHT DOSAGE

When the dosage is not mentioned:

(1) The recommended dosage for fresh juices extracted from herbs is approx. 10 to 20 ml, to be taken twice a day.

(2) The recommended dosage for powders prepared by crushing dried herbs (preferably dried in shade) is approx. 3 to 5 g.

(3) The recommended dosage for a decoction prepared by boiling approx. 10 to 20 g of a particular herb is 50 to 100 ml to be taken lukewarm once or twice a day.

ABBREVIATIONS

tsp - teaspoons   **tbsp** - tablespoons

ml - millilitres   **g** - grams

Contents

Introduction		xiii
1.	Acidity	1
2.	Amoebiasis	3
3.	Asthma	5
4.	Bronchitis	8
5.	Common Cold	11
6.	Constipation	13
7.	Diabetes	15
8.	Diarrhoea	17
9.	Indigestion	19
10.	Obesity	21
11.	Tonsillitis	22
12.	Hoarseness of the Voice	24
13.	Tuberculosis	26
14.	Vomiting	28
15.	Piles	31
16.	Ascites	33
17.	Viral Hepatitis	34
18.	Spleenomegaly	36
19.	Jaundice	38
20.	Gall Bladder Stones	40

21.	Cirrhosis of the Liver	42
22.	Loss of Appetite	44
23.	Urticaria	46
24.	Eczema	47
25.	Leucoderma	49
26.	Acne	51
27.	Boils	53
28.	Hair Loss	55
29.	Osteoarthritis	57
30.	Rheumatoid Arthritis	59
31.	Gout	61
32.	Lumbar Spondylitis	63
33.	Epilepsy	64
34.	Giddiness	66
35.	Sleeplessness	68
36.	Sciatica	70
37.	Anxiety	72
38.	Urinary Tract Infection	73
39.	Urinary Retention	75
40.	Urinary Stones	77
41.	Blood in Urine	79
42.	Renal Colic	81
43.	Prostate Enlargement	82
44.	Bedwetting	84

45.	Leucorrhoea	86
46.	Painful Menstruation	88
47.	Excessive Menstruation	90
48.	Scanty Menstruation	91
49.	Differential Uterine Bleeding	93
50.	Goitre	94
51.	Anaemia	95
52.	Ear Disorders	97
53.	Nose Bleed	99
54.	Fever	101
55.	Gas Trouble	103
56.	Headache	105
57.	Heart Disease	108
58.	High Blood Pressure	110
59.	Uterine Prolapse	111
60.	Mouth Ulcers	113
61.	Worm Infestation	115
62.	Low Blood Pressure	118
63.	Hernia	120
64.	Stomach Ulcer	121
65.	Wound	122
66.	Toothache and Bleeding Gums	124
67.	Decreased Lactation	126
68.	Swelling	128

69.	Depression	130
70.	Sore Throat	132
71.	Whooping Cough	134
72.	Cramps	135
73.	Hiccough	136
74.	Cervical Spondylitis	138
75.	Cough	139
76.	Impotence	141
77.	Hysteria	142
78.	Heat Stroke	144
79.	Dysentery	145
80.	Typhoid	146
81.	Pneumonia	147
82.	Leprosy	148
83.	Sterility	150
84.	Thinness	151
85.	Itching	153
86.	Scabies	154
87.	Measles	155
88.	Mental Ailment	157
89.	Filariasis	159
90.	Diptheria	160
91.	Fungal Infection	162
92.	Ulcerative Colitis	164

93.	Flu	166
94.	Spruce	167
95.	Sore Tongue	169
96.	Haemorrhage	170
97.	Thirst	171
98.	Defective Eyesight	173
99.	Conjunctivitis	175
100.	Greying of Hair	177

INTRODUCTION

While the use of allopathic drugs have increased, an awareness of their harmful side-effects has also risen. People have begun to question the safety and efficacy of mass-produced drugs, and are beginning to turn increasingly to Herbal Remedies. These are becoming easier to find both in India and abroad. They are safe to use and less expensive.

These factors have motivated me to write on the subject of Home Remedies that are harmless and have stood the test of time. They can be used as preventives, or to treat a disease.

The responses that I have received to my articles and the success of my first book, *Herbal Healers*, on this subject have been the testimony that gives me added confidence.

In this book I have listed 100 common diseases, with a brief description of their symptoms and the Ayurvedic view point in each case. This is followed by a list of recommended remedies.

The reader will be encouraged to discover that many of the herbs and spices found in the kitchen have a medicinal value as well. This book aims to be a Guide to Herbs and how and when to use them. It aims to bring Health, Hope and Happiness within our grasp.

Disclaimer: Although every caution has been exercised in compilation of this book, the contents cannot replace medication. These remedies should be taken under medical supervision.

ACIDITY
Ayurdevic Name *Amalpitta*

Characteristic Symptoms

- Acidic eructation and a burning sensation in the chest.
- Loss of hunger or false appetite, nausea, vomiting, weakness and irritation.
- Pain and tenderness in the upper part of the abdomen.
- Aggravated pain on an empty stomach or immediately after taking a meal.
- History of preference for spicy, fried foods, tea, coffee and alcohol.
- Haemorrhage might be seen in chronic cases.

Ayurvedic View

The 5 types are:
1. Caused by vitiation of *vatta* or air body humor.
2. Caused by vitiation of *kapha* or phlegm body humor.
3. Caused by vitiation of both air and phlegm.
4. When there are sour vomits, heartburn and sour eructation, it is called *urdhavag amalpitta*.
5. When there are associated symptoms of greenish or blackish stools along with nausea and vertigo, it is called *adhog amalpitta*.

Management by Home Cures

- The fresh juice extracted from aloe vera is an excellent remedy. Take 20 to 30 ml twice a day, preferably on an empty stomach.

- Take approx. 30 ml of the juice of white pumpkin with some coconut milk and *mishri*, 2 or 3 times a day.
- Take 10 to 20 ml of the juice extracted from the *aamla* fruit on an empty stomach in the morning.
- Add a few drops each of ginger and lemon juice to a glass of warm water; add 1 tsp of honey and take this drink twice a day.
- Mix 1 tsp *isabgol* in a glassful of lukewarm milk and take at bedtime.
- Coconut is beneficial in curing hyperacidity and its associated symptoms like gastritis, excessive thirst and heartburn. Take coconut water 2 or 3 times daily for a few days.
- Take 3 to 5 g powdered *mulathee*, along with cow's milk This is a good cure for acidity and also heals stomach ulcers.
- Try taking an infusion prepared with coriander seeds with some *mishri* added to it.
- Take fresh pomegranate juice in moderate quantities twice a day.

AMOEBIASIS
Ayurvedic Name *Pravahika*

Characteristic Symptoms
- Pain or discomfort in the lower abdomen and recurrent diarrhoea generally alternating with constipation.
- Semisolid stools containing mucous and sometimes blood.
- The causative organism can be found in the fresh stools.

Ayurvedic View
The 4 types are:
1. Caused by vitiation of air body humor.
2. Caused by distortion of the fire humor.
3. Caused by vitiation of the phlegm body humor.
4. Caused by disorders of the blood.

Management by Home Cures
- Take approx. 1 tsp of the dried powder of *bilgiri* (seed of *Aegle marmelos*) mixed with honey, twice a day.
- Mix approx. ½ g powdered nutmeg in buttermilk and take it twice a day.
- Take approx. 5 to 10 ml of the juice extracted from the juvenile leaflets and flowers of *neem* once or twice a day.
- Take the pulp of the fruit of *bael* mixed with some jaggery.
- Take an infusion of lemon on an empty stomach.
- Mix the powder of *isabgol* with yoghurt (curd) and some roasted cumin seeds. Take this 2 or 3 times a day.

- Mix the powdered seeds of henna with a little ghee and take it twice.
- For chronic amoebiasis, roast the pulp of the unripe fruit of *bael* and mix it with an equal quantity of dried ginger powder. Take this with buttermilk 2 or 3 times.
- Take *jamun* preparations or eat the fruit during the season.
- The seeds of *isabgol*, when roasted, tend to bind the loose stools and are recommended as a treatment.
- Take the powder prepared from the dried flowers of the mango tree.

ASTHMA
Ayurvedic Name *Tamak Shwas*

Characteristic Symptoms
- Difficulty in breathing and a feeling of constriction and tightening around the chest.
- A wheezing sound is produced when the breath is expelled.
- During the process of recurrent attacks, the patient feels suffocated.
- There is forward fighting for the breath, a prolonged expiration, and a short and gasping inspiration.
- Bouts of coughing along with tenacious and mucoid sputum.
- In chronic cases, the face turns pale and the body emaciated.

Ayurvedic View
According to Ayurveda, asthma originates from an affliction of the stomach and the gastro-intestinal tract. This can be confirmed from the fact that in the initial stages of the disease the patient shows signs of indigestion accompanied by diarrhoea or constipation, though the main affected organ is the lung. Constant pressure on the lungs even affects the heart. Therefore, while treating the disease, proper attention is given to the working of the stomach, bowels, lungs, nasal region as well as the heart in chronic cases.

Management by Home Cures

- It is of prime importance to become aware of the allergens that trigger the symptoms, and try to avoid them.
- Take 1 tsp turmeric powder twice a day along with warm water.
- Prepare a decoction by boiling equal parts of ginger, holy basil and black pepper. Take this mixed with ½ tsp honey.
- Prepare a powder from dried and pounded black pepper, ginger and *pippali*. Take 1 tsp of the powder along with warm water, twice a day. This helps to relieve the bronchial spasm.
- Take 1 tsp honey and a few drops of ginger juice on an empty stomach in the morning.
- Inhale the fumes produced by boiling some *ajwain* in water. This helps relieve chest congestion.
- In bronchial asthma, when phlegm remains stuck in the bronchioles, *ajwain* helps to reduce the excessive production of phlegm. Take it in the form of powder twice daily, or make a decoction with *ajwain* and take it warm.
- The smoke that results from burning *hing* can be inhaled to get relief from spasms of bronchial asthma.
- Being antiseptic in nature and a destroyer of phlegm, betel leaves are used for treating bronchial asthma. Mix approx. 5 to 10 ml of the juice extracted from betel leaves with freshly ground basil, mint and ginger. Add about 4 to 5 freshly pounded peppercorns to the paste.

Take ½ tsp of this preparation twice a day, along with some honey.
- Add 2 or 3 cloves of garlic to a glassful of milk. Boil for some time and drink it hot.
- Mint is also recommended as a home cure for asthma as it has the property of decreasing phlegm. Extract some juice by crushing fresh mint leaves and add an equal quantity of ginger juice. Take 5 to 10 ml of this mixture twice a day, along with honey.
- *Tulsi* contains specific anti-asthmatic properties. Extract fresh juice by pounding some *tulsi* leaves and take the juice twice a day. Add a few drops of ginger and some honey to build resistance against the disease.

BRONCHITIS

Ayurvedic Name *Shwas Pranali Shoth*

Characteristic Symptoms

- Inflammation of the bronchi of the lungs.
- Initially there is an irritating, dry cough along with chest pain or discomfort.
- Later the cough is persistent and productive with mucoid, viscous or blood-streaked sputum.
- A sensation of tightness in the chest, difficulty in taking a breath, and wheezing sounds.
- Mild to moderate fever, malaise and sore throat.

Ayurvedic View

Five types of bronchitis have been identified in Ayurvedic texts:

a. Vitiation of *vatta* or the air body humor causes its movement towards the upper part of the head and neck, and produces a cough which sounds like torn bamboo.

b. Caused by vitiation in the *pitta* or fire humor.

c. Caused by vitiation of *kapha* or phlegm humor.

d. Owing to external factors the distorted air causes an injury in the chest region and the cough is accompanied with blood.

e. Owing to impairment of digestion, an imbalance in all the three humors causes the disease or it may be a consequence of tuberculosis.

Management by Home Cures

- Take 1 tsp turmeric powder along with warm water, once or twice a day.
- Grind dried ginger, black pepper and long pepper together in equal quantities and take this twice with honey.
- Extract the juice from the leaves of *vasa* and take 1 to 2 tsp along with honey.
- For chronic bronchitis, a decoction prepared from the herbs *vasa, vacha, pipali* and *mulethi* is very effective. Take approx. 20 to 30 ml, warmed, twice a day.
- Roast approx. 1 tsp *ajwain* and pound into a powder; add double the amount of powdered *mishri* and take with warm water twice or thrice a day.
- In bronchitis, local massage of a warm paste of *hing* on the chest also proves useful.
- Betel leaf is another herb that is helpful if you are suffering from bronchitis or chronic cough. As a home remedy try mixing approx.
  5 to 10 ml juice extracted from betel leaves with freshly ground basil, mint and ginger. Add about 4 to 5 pounded peppercorns to the paste. Take ½ tsp of this preparation twice, along with some honey. Gargle with the juice extracted from betel leaves.
- For acute as well as chronic bronchitis you will benefit with regular use of ginger. Add a few drops of the juice to your daily tea and keep away the disease.
- Suck on 2 to 4 black peppercorns 2 or 3 times a day and swallow the juice slowly.

- The leaves of basil act as an expectorant and help in removing phlegm. The juice of the leaves of basil is recommended in the treatment of bronchitis.
- For a chronic cough and bronchitis take garlic juice regularly, extracted by pounding a few bulbs of garlic.
- Take approx. 1 to 3 g powdered cinnamon mixed in 1 tsp honey. For better relief add a pinch of black pepper powder and a few drops of ginger juice.
- Pound the leaves and extract the juice of henna; take ½ tsp, 2 times a day, mixed in an equal quantity of honey. You could also try to gargle with a decoction of henna leaves.

COMMON COLD
Ayurvedic Name *Pratishaya*

Characteristic Symptoms
- Abrupt onset along with tickling sensation in the nasal tract.
- Running nose, sneezing and obstruction of nasal passage.
- Pharyngeal and conjunctival itching.
- Malaise, headache, dryness and soreness of throat.
- Spread of the infection may result in earache, bronchitis or pneumonia.

Ayurvedic View
Five types of cold or *Pratishaya* have been specified:
a. Caused by vitiation of air body humor.
b. Caused by vitiation of the fire body humor.
c. Caused by vitiation of the phlegm body humor.
d. Chronic cold caused by all the three humors.
e. Caused by the disorders of the blood.

Management by Home Cures
- Steam inhalation by burning a piece of turmeric can provide instant relief from a running nose.
- Gargle with saline water or warm water with a pinch of *phitkari* added to it, 3 to 4 times a day.
- For relief from nasal block, make a powder by pounding together black peppercorns, cardamom, cinnamon and black cumin seeds in equal parts and sniff it.

- Pound approx. 6 g of garlic with an equal quantity of jaggery. Take this at bedtime.
- Mix approx. 5 to 10 ml juice extracted from betel leaves with freshly ground basil, mint and ginger. Add about 4 to 5 pounded peppercorns to the paste. Take ½ tsp of this preparation twice, mixed into some honey.
- Pound some fresh leaves of *bilva* to extract their juice and take approx. 10 to 20 ml, 2 to 3 times.
- Prepare a decoction with ginger, basil and pepper. Take it warm twice a day mixed with ½ tsp honey.
- During the first stage of a cold, when you are bound to suffer from continuous watery discharge from the nose, try this: Boil ½ tsp black pepper powder in a glassful of milk and take it warm at bedtime.
- External massage of a paste of *hing* on the chest helps.
- Catechu tends to cause decrease in phlegm or kapha body humor, making it a useful remedy for the common cold. Take ½ to 1 g Catechu twice a day, mixed with honey.
- Put 2-3 drops of ghee in the nostrils as nasal drops once or twice a day.
- Cinnamon is also a destroyer of phlegm and is recommended in treating a cold. Take approx 1 to 3 g cinnamon powder mixed with 1 tsp honey. For better relief add a pinch of black pepper powder and a few drops of ginger juice.
- Pound the leaves of henna to extract the juice and take ½ tsp, 2 times a day. Preferably mix the juice into an equal quantity of honey.

CONSTIPATION

Ayurvedic Name *Vibandh, Kostha Badhata, Aanah*

Characteristic Symptoms

- Delay in frequency of the bowels, hard stools, a feeling of incomplete evacuation and pain and difficulty in passing stools.
- Heaviness in the stomach, abdominal cramps, increased wind formation, headache, dizziness, lethargy, loss of appetite and sometimes bleeding while defecating.

Ayurvedic View

Two types have been specified:
a. Caused by accumulation of undigested food juice called *aamaj aanah*.
b. Caused by accumulation of waste matter in the intestines, called *purishaj aanah*.

Management by Home Cures

- Take 2 heaped tsp *isabgol* powder once in the daytime and once at bedtime with warm milk or water. The better way is to add approx. 1 glassful of water or milk to the husk of *isabgol*; let it soak for at least 1 to 2 hours; take preferably at bedtime. It is desirable to add some sugar to the *isabgol* preparation.
- Fry *harad* in ghee, then powder it. Take this along with warm water once or twice daily for a few days.
- Make a powder by crushing the leaves of senna and take ½ tsp twice with warm water.

- Mix 1 tsp ghee in a cup of warm milk and take this at bedtime regularly for some days.
- Take powdered *mulathi* mixed with jaggery to relieve constipation.
- Extract the pulp from the roots of *arni*, roast it in ghee and take it with warm milk.
- Soak some black raisins in hot water for a few hours then mash them and drink the juice, preferably at bedtime.
- Mix 1 to 2 tsp purified castor oil and ¼ tsp dried ginger powder in a cup of warm water and take at bedtime.
- Take 1 to 2 tsp sweet rose jelly called *gulkanda* twice, along with warm milk.
- Roast and powder fennel. In case of habitual constipation, try taking it with warm milk at bedtime.
- Soak a few dates in milk till soft; mash their pulp and mix in milk. Take it twice for a few days.
- Mix 1 to 2 tsp pure castor oil with warm milk and take it at bedtime.
- Take approx. 3 to 5 g of the powder of *harad* along with warm water to get relief from constipation.
- For small children and babies with constipation and abdominal gas, a home remedy is to make them lick a pinch of the powder of *harad* along with some honey.
- As a home remedy for habitual constipation, take 1 tsp honey in lukewarm water on an empty stomach regularly. This clears the bowels and acts as a prophylactic against the problems of digestion.
- Take equal quantities of turmeric powder and black salt along with warm water after meals.

DIABETES
Ayurvedic Name *Madhumeha*

Characteristic Symptoms
- Increased frequency of urination; large amounts of urine; low specific gravity of urine; excessive thirst and general body weakness.
- There may be signs of diabetic degeneration, delay or non-healing of wounds and muscle wasting.

Ayurvedic View
Twenty types of *prameha* have been specified in Ayurvedic texts:

a. Caused by vitiation of *vatta* or air body humor; there are 4 varieties that are considered incurable.

b. Caused by vitiation of *pitta* or fire body humor; there are 6 varieties that are difficult to cure.

c. Caused by vitiation of *kapha* or phlegm body humor; there are 10 varieties that are considered curable.

Management by Home Cures
- Pound the seeds of *karela* and take 3 to 5 g of the powder twice along with warm water.
- Extract the juice by grinding fresh *karela*. Take the juice on an empty stomach.
- Pound together the tender leaves of *neem* and *bilva* and roll into small balls. Take 2 to 4 of these along with warm water first thing in the morning on an empty stomach.

- *Bilva* has the property of reducing the blood sugar levels and abating excessive urination. Take approx. 20 ml of the juice extracted from *bilva* leaves. On an empty stomach the benefits are greater.
- *Brahmi* is pungent and astringent and is believed to be helpful in diabetes. Patients are advised to supplement their routine therapy with this herbal preparation.
- *Jamun* is useful in the treatment of diabetes. Prepare a powder by crushing the dried seeds of the fruit. Take 1 tsp of the powder to supplement your routine medication.
- Extract the juice from a few juvenile leaves of the mango tree and take it with an equal quantity of the juice of *karela* on an empty stomach during the initial stages of the disease.
- It is advisable for diabetic patients to chew 3 to 5 fresh leaves of *neem* on an empty stomach first thing in the morning. The *neem* oil and resin extracted from the bark are also recommended. Being pungent, it also relieves excessive urination.
- It is beneficial for diabetics to take the fresh juice of *aamla* on an empty stomach.
- The flour of groundnut is also believed to be beneficial. Make chappatis with groundnut flour mixed with wheat flour.

DIARRHOEA
Ayurvedic Name *Atisaar*

Characteristic Symptoms
- Looseness of bowels and an increase in frequency and fluidity of stools.
- The stools turn copious and more in volume.

Ayurvedic View
Six types of diarrhoea or *atisaar* have been specified:
a. Caused by vitiation of the air body humor.
b. Caused by vitiation of the fire body humor.
c. Caused by vitiation of the phlegm body humor.
d. Caused by vitiation of all the three body humors: air, fire and phlegm.
e. Caused by mental states of grief, etc.
f. Caused by indigestion of the previous meal.

Management by Home Cures
- Extract the pulp of the fruit of *bilva* and roast it. Mix it with an equal quantity of jaggery and take it twice a day.
- Make an infusion with the bark of *babool* and take it every 6 hours.
- Pound the dried seeds of *bael* into a powder. Take 3 to 5 g with water 2 or 3 times.
- Take 1 to 3 g of the powdered seeds of henna; these have the tendency to bind stools.

- Pound nutmeg, dried ginger, seeds of *bael* and *atis* into a powder. Take approx. ¼ tsp of this powdered mixture twice with water.
- The roasted seeds of *isabgol* bind loose stools and are recommended.
- Take equal quantities of dried ginger powder and powdered rock salt. Mix ¼ tsp of the mixture into some jaggery and take this twice a day.
- Take 3 to 6 g of the powder of the dried seeds of *jamun* in chronic diarrhoea.
- Roast the kernel of the mango fruit. Pound it into a powder and take it with lemon juice and black salt.
- Take a powder prepared from the dried flowers of the mango tree.
- In the cases of non-specific diarrhoea, mint can be used because mint contains anti-toxic properties. Prepare a paste by pounding together Mint leaves and onions and take 1 to 2 tsp of this paste 3 to 4 times a day.
- Nutmeg binds loose stools and reduces the after-effects, like weakness, loss of taste, and fever. Powder nutmeg and take ½ to 1 gram twice a day along with water or buttermilk.

INDIGESTION
Ayurvedic Name *Ajiran, Agnimandhya*

Characteristic Symptoms
- Pain in the upper abdomen; belching; excessive wind formation; abdominal distension; false hunger; nausea and vomiting.
- Off and on changes in the bowels.
- Sometimes heartburn and a continuous feeling of discomfort.

Ayurvedic View
Six types of the disease have been specified:
a. Caused by vitiation of *vatta* or air body humor called *vishtabdha ajiran*.
b. Caused by vitiation of *pitta* or fire humor called *vidagdha ajiran*.
c. Caused by vitiation of the phlegm or *kapha* called *aama ajiran*.
d. When the meal is not digested properly, *rasshesha* ajiran results.
e. When it takes the whole day to digest the meal, this is *dinpaki* ajiran.
f. Sometimes there is natural indigestion of the previous meal; this is *prakrit ajiran*.

Management by Home Cures
- Chew a piece of ginger mixed with powdered rock salt before each meal.
- Buttermilk mixed with powdered *hing* and black salt can be taken 3 or 4 times a day.

- Mix lemon juice with a pinch each of powdered black pepper, roasted cumin seeds and black salt and take 2 or 3 times.
- Take a mixture of equal quantities of powdered dried ginger, rock salt and black pepper, along with a glass of warm water, before meals.
- Pound the seeds of large cardamom and take approx. 1 to 3 g of the powder, preferably with some warm water.
- The juice of *karela*, even in small quantities, alleviates indigestion.
- Add the juice of one-fourth of a freshly cut lemon to a glass of lukewarm water and also add a mixture of equal quantities of powdered black pepper, cumin seeds, dry coriander, thyme and black salt. Take 2 or 3 times a day.
- Take equal quantities of ginger and lime juice (approx. 1 tsp). To this add a pinch each of black salt and black pepper. Take it twice with warm water after meals.
- Take approx. 2 to 3 tsp of the juice extracted by pounding freshly cut onions, mixed with a pinch of turmeric on an empty stomach.
- A small quantity of freshly pounded black pepper with some buttermilk gives quick relief.
- Pound a piece of cinnamon and boil in a glass of water. Take this drink lukewarm at least half an hour before meals.
- A decoction prepared by boiling equal parts of fennel and thyme seeds is particularly beneficial for small babies who have indigestion.
- Take the leaves of mint, either in raw form or made into chutney.

OBESITY

Ayurvedic Name *Aatisthoola, Medho Vridhi*

Characteristic Symptoms
- Excessive increase in body fat and body weight.
- Fatty and bulky body stature.
- The patient is usually lethargic, inactive and obsessed.
- Increased skin-fold thickness over the triceps muscle.

Ayurvedic View
Ayurveda believes that the actual cause of obesity is the impairment of the gastric fire or *agni* responsible for breaking up the molecules of fat.

Management by Home Cures
- Soak *trifla* powder overnight in water. Take this on an empty stomach first thing in the morning, continuously for some days. To make it more beneficial, add ½ to 1 tsp honey.
- Mix ½ tsp honey in a glass of warm water along with a few drops of lemon and take it in the morning.
- Take approx 15 grains of pure *guggul*, 2 or 3 times along with hot water.
- Dry massage of the entire body should be practiced daily; a massage with mustard oil is helpful.
- Mix groundnut flour into wheat flour and make into chappatis.
- Taking 1 to 2 grams of *shilajit* per day may be of help. This can be continued for a few days.
- Add pure *shilajit* to *guggul* and pound together. Take this mixture twice a day.

TONSILLITIS
Ayurvedic Name *Tundikeri Shoth*

Characteristic Symptoms
- Pain in the throat that increases on swallowing.
- The pain generally radiates to the ear.
- High grade fever; malaise; loss of hunger; dry and irritant cough; excessive thirst and feeling of chill.
- Tonsils become swollen, engorged and sometimes congested.

Ayurvedic View
Vitiation in any of the three body humors - air, fire and phlegm, or in all three is the cause the disease.

Management by Home Cures
- Prepare a decoction by boiling a few leaves of basil, ginger and cloves. Take 20 ml, warmed, with 1 tsp honey, twice or thrice a day.
- Gargle with a decoction prepared by boiling the bark of the acacia tree.
- Mix approx. 1 tsp of each of the powders of *mulathi* and *vacha* into honey. Take twice or thrice a day.
- Gargle with warm black tea with some salt added to it to get relief.
- Boil approx. 15 g of the flowers of *banafsha* in 50 ml milk. Take warm twice a day. The filtered residue can be heated and tied around the throat in the form of a poultice.

- Take honey regularly for preventing as well as for curing tonsillitis.
- Gargle with warm water boiled with some *tulsi* leaves.
- The milk from a raw papaya can be applied on the inflamed tonsils like throat paint.
- Dissolve powdered *phitkari* in water and use as a gargle.
- Gargle with warmed lemon water.

HOARSENESS OF THE VOICE
Ayurvedic Name *Swarbheda*

Characteristic Symptoms
- Inflammation of the larynx or the voice box caused by infection, abnormal growth or by taking hot and cold substances alternately.
- Change of voice and difficulty in vocalisation.
- Dry, irritating cough, pain in swallowing and a persistent urge to clear the throat.
- A coated tongue, a tickling or burning sensation in the throat and fever.

Ayurvedic View
Swarbheda is generally believed to result from inflammation of the larynx. This may be as a consequence of vitiation in the body humors due to an abnormal growth, taking hot and cold substances alternately, infection by a micro-organism or an infection produced by chronic tuberculosis.

Management by Home Cures
- Chew (masticate) some black pepper and *mishri* because the juice eases the hoarseness.
- Gargle with the juice of wheat grass and also drink it.
- Prepare a decoction by boiling the bark of the acacia tree and use it for gargling.
- Take approx. 1 tsp each of the powders of *vacha* and *yashtimadhu* with honey twice daily to get relief.

- Gargling with *phitkari* mixed with water is quite helpful.
- Suck on a piece of *catechu* as a lozenge.
- Gargle with water in which some *catechu* powder has been boiled.
- Roast a piece of the dried fruit of *baheda*. Keep it in your mouth and slowly suck the juice.

TUBERCULOSIS
Ayurvedic Name *Rajyakshma, Kshaya Roga*

Characteristic Symptoms
- Loss of weight; loss of appetite and general malaise.
- Rising temperature in the evenings; night sweats and recurrent bouts of cough.
- The cough lasts for more than 3 weeks and remains unexplained.
- Pain in the chest and sometimes blood in the sputum.

Ayurvedic View
According to the Ayurvedic theory, this disease arises as a consequence of an imbalance of all the three humors of the body: air, fire and phlegm. This leads to blocking of the *srotas* or the various channels and later the emaciation of the *dhatus* or the body tissues, resulting in tuberculosis.

Management by Home Cures
- Extract the juice by crushing the fresh fruit of *aamla* and take approx 20 ml twice with 1 tsp honey.
- Mix approx. 1 tsp each of the powders of *vacha* and liquorice in honey or warm water and take it twice.
- Cinnamon combats phlegm and it has been researched that Cinnamic acid has anti-tubercular properties. Take 1 to 3 grams of powdered cinnamom along with warm water twice a day.
- Both the external as well as internal use of cloves reduces the vitiation of both the fire and phlegm body humors.

- In Ayurvedic therapy, intake as well as local application of coconut oil is recommended in treating tuberculosis.
- Prepare a decoction by boiling equal parts of garlic and *vayavidanga*. Take the decoction and also apply externally on the chest.
- Grapes are recommended as they are exceptionally strengthening for the lungs and are also an expectorant.
- The flour of groundnut can be included in the daily diet.
- The bark of the *neem* tree contains an oily substance which is believed to be useful in treating tuberculosis. Prepare a decoction with the bark and take approx. ½ cup twice daily.

VOMITING

Ayurvedic Name   *Chhardi, Vaman*

Characteristic Symptoms

- Forceful expulsion of the gastric contents through the mouth.
- The contents of the vomit may have food particles, bile, water or even blood.
- The presence of blood reveals bleeding from the stomach, small intestine or the food pipe.
- Dehydration may result in extreme cases.
- The cause may be intake of toxic food, pregnancy, intestinal worms or mental illness.

Ayurvedic View

Five types of *chhardi roga* have been specified in Ayurvedic texts:

a. Caused by vitiation of the air body humor.
b. Caused by vitiation of the fire humor.
c. Caused by vitiation of the phlegm humor.
d. Caused by vitiation of all the 3 humors, *vatta, pitta* and *kapha*.
e. Caused by worm infestations or unpleasant sights, smells, touches, tastes and sounds.

Management by Home Cures

- Take the ashes of small cardamoms mixed with honey.
- Slowly suck a piece of lemon or ice.
- Take 1.125 g ashes of a peacock feather twice or thrice a day along with water or mixed into honey.

- Burn the bark of the peepul tree; then extinguish it in water. Strain this water in a linen cloth and take it every 6 to 8 hours to get relief.
- Simply chew 1 or 2 cardamoms and slowly swallow the juice.
- Make a decoction by boiling cardamoms along with some mint leaves; add some *mishri*. Take in small quantities at regular intervals. In case of children, pound cardamoms and make them lick the powder mixed in a little honey.
- Make a paste of parched rice diluted in water; add the powders of cloves and cardamom and some sugar.
- In case of nausea or vomiting, take equal quantities of powdered fennel and dried mint leaves. Boil these in water till one-fourth remains. Take this decoction 3 to 4 times a day.
- A decoction prepared by boiling equal parts of fennel and thyme seeds is particularly beneficial for small babies in treating vomiting and indigestion.
- Pound the fresh, juvenile leaves of *jamun* to extract the juice. Take 10 to 20 ml to treat nausea and vomiting.
- You could take a lemon drink supplemented with a generous amount of sugar. Or simply lick a freshly sliced lemon. This is quite useful during the nausea associated with travelling.
- Another easy home remedy is to peel the lemon skin and dry it; burn the skin and collect the ashes. Take the ashes with some water to find relief.

- Pound mint leaves and onions together to make a paste. Take 1 to 2 tsp of the paste 3 to 4 times a day.
- Suck on 2 or 3 cloves.
- To the freshly extracted juice of *tulsi*, add equal quantities of the juice of mint and ginger; for better results you can add a little *saunf arka* as well. Take this mixture every 4 hours for relief.

PILES
Ayurvedic Name *Arsh Roga*

Characteristic Symptoms
- The veins in the anal region become varicose.
- In dry or external piles, there is an inflammation of the external veins. Pain is a regular feature which becomes unbearable while passing stools.
- In case of bleeding piles or internal haemorrhoids, the internal veins are enlarged and inflammed. Sometimes there is excessive bleeding which results in anaemia, discomfort and general weakness. The blood is generally unmixed with stools.
- There may be a prolapse of the rectum.

Ayurvedic View
Five types of *arsh roga* have been stated:
a. Caused by vitiation of air body humor.
b. Caused by vitiation of fire body humor.
c. Caused by vitiation of phlegm body humor.
d. Caused by vitiation of any 2 body humors.
e. Caused by vitiation of all the 3 humors, air, fire and phlegm.

Management by Home Cures
- Take 3 to 5 g of the powder of *harad* twice with water or milk.
- Keep approx. ½ g of camphor in a piece of banana and take it in the morning on an empty stomach. You could

repeat this remedy for 2 or 3 days both for dry as well as bleeding piles.
- Apply a poultice prepared from *haridra* and *vijaya*.
- Make a powder by pounding the dried flowers of *nagakesar* and take 1 to 3 g approx. with honey 2 or 3 times to find relief.
- Soak 2 to 3 figs in a glass of water overnight. In the morning mash them in the water and take the drink on an empty stomach. Repeat for a few days.
- The raw fruit of *bilva* tends to arrest blood loss; therefore, in maladies where there is loss of blood from the body like bleeding piles, *bilva* formulations are a drug of choice. As a home remedy for these ailments, roast the pulp extracted from the raw fruit of *bilva*; remove and mix into an equal quantity of jaggery and take 2 or 3 times.
- For bleeding piles, take a glass of warm cow's milk and mix into the juice extracted from half a lemon. Drink immediately. Repeat once for 2 or 3 days.
- For bleeding piles, take sesame seeds mixed with some butter. Sesame has the property of stopping blood loss. A paste made by pounding sesame seeds can also be applied on the haemorrhoids for relief.
- Apply a paste made by grinding radish in milk at the site of piles.
- Take the fresh juice of *aamla* on an empty stomach.
- For bleeding piles you could try this remedy: Take approx. 1 to 3 g of the powder prepared by pounding the dried pollen of *nagkeshar* along with milk or water twice a day.

ASCITES
Ayurvedic Name *Jalodar*

Characteristic Symptoms
- Accumulation of free fluid in the abdomen.
- Rigidity and tenderness in the right or upper side of the abdomen.
- Normally associated with a liver disease like cirrhosis.

Ayurvedic View

This disease is believed to result from distortion of the gastric fire which may be caused by excessive intake of water by an emaciated person, or a person having a weak digestion, or a normal person taking water after the intake of oily and fatty foods. When this water combines with vitiated phlegm body humor, it causes this disease.

Management by Home Cures
- Prepare a decoction by boiling the roots of *punarnava*: Take approx 30 ml at least twice daily.
- Take 120 mg of the powder of *kutaki* once or twice a day along with warm water.
- Pound the dried roots of *punarnava* to make a powder. Take approx.
  1 tsp twice along with lukewarm water.
- Prepare a powder by pounding together the 3 *myrobalans* (*aamla*, *harad* and *baheda*) in equal quantities and take 1 tsp along with a decoction of *punarnava* roots or the *arka* of *punarnava*.

VIRAL HEPATITIS
Ayurvedic Name   *Yakrit Shoth*

Characteristic Symptoms
- Pain in the upper, right part of the abdomen.
- Nausea, vomiting, malaise, loss of hunger and low-grade fever may occur.
- Clay-coloured stools and dark urine begin to be seen, subsequently followed by clinical jaundice.

Ayurvedic View
It is believed that when a person suffering from anaemia takes those foodstuffs in large quantities which tend to aggravate the *pitta dosha* or heat body humor, then the increased heat burns the blood and muscle *dhatus* or body tissues. This causes hepatitis.

Management by Home Cures
- Extract the fresh juice from the pulp of aloe vera and take approx.
  10 to 20 ml twice a day on an empty stomach.
- Crush the rhizome of *kutaki* to make a powder. Take approx. 1 g of the powder twice along with some warm water.
- Soak approx. 100 g of dried tamarind and 50 g of plums in water overnight. In the morning mash the ingredients, add some black salt and drink this thick liquid.
- Pound *bhui aamlaki* into a paste and mix it into some buttermilk. Take this preferably on an empty stomach.

- Extract the juice from white onions and mix approx. 2 to 3 tbsp with ¼ tsp turmeric powder and some sugar. Take it twice a day.
- Pound the herb *bhringraj* and extract the juice. Take approx. 20 ml twice.

SPLEENOMEGALY
Ayurvedic Name *Pleehodar*

Characteristic Symptoms
- Enlargement of the spleen generally caused by some chronic ailment.
- The causative disorder could be typhoid, malaria, hepatitis, anaemia, syphilis, rheumatoid arthritis, leukaemia, lymphoma, tuberculosis, etc.
- Acute pain in the left abdominal region.
- Perhaps mild fever and anaemia.
- General weakness and debility.

Ayurvedic View
The phlegm humor of the body combines with impure blood and causes this disease. It is of three types:

a. Caused by vitiation in the air body humor or *vatta*. The symptoms are pain, fullness in the abdomen and excessive wind formation.

b. Caused by vitiation of *pitta* or fire. Excessive thirst, fever and a burning sensation are the dominant symptoms.

c. Caused by distortion of phlegm or *kapha*. The main symptoms are loss of appetite, heaviness and rigidity.

Management by Home Cures
- Take approx. 1 g of the powder of *kutaki* twice a day with honey or buttermilk.
- Take 20 ml of the fresh juice of aloe vera twice.

- Prepare a decoction by boiling flowers of *shalmali*. Take 10 to 20 ml thrice a day.
- Prepare a powder by pounding 2 to 4 g of the seeds of mustard. Take this twice a day. Local massage of mustard oil on the region of the enlarged spleen is also advised. This 'mustard therapy' is believed to be quite helpful in treating this ailment.
- Mix some turmeric powder in the pulp of aloe vera, heat the mixture on low heat then tie it in a cloth and put it on the site of the enlarged spleen.

JAUNDICE
Ayurvedic Name *Kamla*

Characteristic Symptoms
- Yellow colouration of the skin, sclera and the mucous membrane of the mouth.
- Dark urine and pale - coloured stools.
- The underlying cause can be either damage of the liver cells due to an infection, inflammation of the bile duct due to presence of gallstones, or destruction of a large quantity of red blood cells.
- Tender, enlarged liver.
- Pain and tenderness in the right, upper part of the abdomen.

Ayurvedic View
When a person suffering from anaemia takes those foodstuffs in large quantities that aggravate the *pitta dosha* or heat body humor, then the increased heat burns the blood and muscle *dhatu* and causes this disease.

Management by Home Cures
- Pound the rhizome *kutaki* to make a powder. Take 1 g of the powder twice with warm water.
- Take approx. 15 to 20 ml of the juice of radish thrice a day.
- Soak approx. 100 g dried tamarind and 50 g plums in water overnight. In the morning mash the ingredients, add some black salt and drink this thick liquid.

- Extract fresh juice from aloe vera. Take approx. 20 ml twice on an empty stomach.
- Extract the fresh juice from the leaves of henna. To 5 to 10 ml of the juice, add a moderate quantity of *mishri* or sugar and take this twice on an empty stomach.
- Pound *bhui aamlaki* into a paste, mix it into buttermilk and take it preferably on an empty stomach.
- Prepare a powder by pounding the 3 *myrobalans*; soak approx. 5 g in water overnight. Mash it and take this first thing in the morning on an empty stomach. You could add 1 tsp honey.
- Extract the juice from white onions and mix approx. 2 to 3 tbsp with ¼ tsp turmeric powder and some sugar. Take it twice a day.
- Pound *bhringraj* and extract the juice. Take approx 20 ml of the juice, twice.
- Pound fresh leaves of spinach to extract the juice and take it 2 or 3 times.
- In our ancient therapies, the juice of sugarcane has been advocated as a treatment of jaundice. Sugarcane tends to improve the working of the liver and acts as a strength booster.
- Pound *giloy* and extract the juice. Take approx 20 ml of this juice twice daily.
- Take 10 to 20 ml of the juice of *karela* twice, preferably on an empty stomach.

GALL BLADDER STONES
Ayurvedic Names *Pittashaya Ashmari*

Characteristic Symptoms
- Pain and discomfort in the upper part of the abdomen, followed by tenderness and rigidity in the right hypochondrium.
- There may be nausea, vomiting, and sometimes fever with chills.
- Pain is aggravated on taking a fatty meal.

Ayurvedic View
Vitiation in the *vatta*, *pitta* and *kapha doshas* of the body cause this disease. The predominant factor is the aggravation in the fire or the *pitta* body humor.

Management by Home Cures
- Pound a few fresh leaves of *patharchat* and take them 2 to 3 times a day.
- Take approx 20 ml of the juice of aloe vera twice on an empty stomach.
- Soak approx. 50 g of the pulse *kulthi* in water overnight. In the morning mash and drink it.
- You could also take 30 ml of the decoction of *kulthi* seeds twice a day.
- Take approx. 1 kg lemon juice. Add approx. 250 g powder of *kaudis* (Calcium carbonate). Leave for a few days. Take 1 tsp of the mixture daily for one month.
- Coconut water may be taken daily 3 or 4 times.

- Pound the root of papaya, extract the juice and mix it with some water. Drink this in the morning on an empty stomach for a few days.

CIRRHOSIS OF THE LIVER
Ayurvedic Name *Yakrit Vishamayta*

Characteristic Symptoms
- Varied symptoms like loss of hunger, nausea, vomiting, fatigue, flatulence, abdominal discomfort, diarrhoea or constipation.
- There may be jaundice, weight loss, swelling, ascites, clubbing of the fingers, splenomegaly, enlargement of the parotid gland, menstrual abnormality.
- Perhaps muscle wasting, nose bleeds and gastro-intestinal bleeding in severe cases.
- The liver is generally firm and nodular.

Ayurvedic View
This disease is believed to be similar to splenomegaly except that the pain is on the right side of the abdomen. The phlegm or *kapha* humor of the body combines with impure blood and causes this disease. It is of three types:
a. Caused by vitiation in the air body humor or *vatta*.
b. Caused by vitiation of *pitta* or the fire body humor.
c. Caused by distortion of phlegm or *kapha*.

Management by Home Cures
- Take approx. 15 ml fresh juice of *bhringraj* twice.
- The fruit of *jamun* tones up the liver and improves its working.
- Take 15-20 ml juice of aloe vera twice on an empty stomach.

- Take approx. 2 to 3 g powdered *methi* along with warm water to tone up a sluggish liver.
- Take 1 g of the powder of the dried rhizome of *kutaki* with warm water twice a day.
- Pound the fresh herbs *punarnava* and *bhui aamla*, and the bark of the *shyonak* tree to extract the juice. Take equal parts (approx. 25 g) once or twice on an empty stomach.
- The juice of *karela*, if taken even in small quantities, could work wonders to improve as well as regulate the working of the liver.
- Pound *punarnava* to extract the juice. Take approx. 20 ml, 2 or 3 times.

LOSS OF APPETITE
Ayurvedic Name *Aruchi*

Characteristic Symptoms
- Anorexia (loss of appetite) is the loss of interest in food, which is generally a symptom in a number of gastro-intestinal diseases.
- Sometimes the cause is an emotional disturbance.

Ayurvedic View
A variety of causes like mental anxiety, fear, anger, greed and dislike for particular foods etc., cause the humors of the body to get vitiated; these further distort the stomach and cause this disease.

Five types of *aruchi* have been specified:
a. Caused by vitiation of *vatta* or air.
b. Caused by vitiation of *pitta* or fire.
c. Caused by vitiation of the phlegm or *kapha* body humor.
d. Caused by a distortion in all the 3 humors.
e. Caused by mental disease. This is called *aaguntaj aaruchi*.

Management by Home Cures
- Take the juice of fresh pomegranates with a pinch of black salt twice.
- The sweet, sour and salty drink called *jal jeera* can be taken 3 to 4 times.
- A small quantity of black pepper powder along with some buttermilk will give quick relief.

- Another easy remedy is to sprinkle some lemon juice on a piece of fresh ginger and take it before a meal.
- Supplement your meals with the leaves of mint, either in raw or chutney form as they are extremely beneficial if you are suffering from loss of appetite.
- Prepare a decoction by boiling mint leaves, basil leaves, ginger, a large cardamom, a pinch of *hing* and some crushed black pepper. Take 20 to 30 ml mixed with some *mishri* or honey 2 to 3 times.
- Chew sesame seeds before meals.

URTICARIA
Ayurvedic Name *Sheetpitta*

Characteristic Symptoms
- Intense itching and burning sensation on the skin.
- This is followed by formation of wheals or swelling on the skin.
- In severe conditions, there may be diffused swelling of the mucous membrane of the mouth and throat leading to respiratory distress involving the upper respiratory tract.

Ayurvedic View
An aggravation of the *vatta* and *kapha* humors of the body in conjugation with vitiation of the *pitta dosha* is believed to cause the disease.

Management by Home Cures
- Local massage of camphor mixed with coconut oil could help relieve the constant itch.
- Mix the seeds of *charonjee* with honey. Take 1 tsp, 2 to 3 times.
- Take ginger in the form of fresh juice (5 to 10 ml) or dried ginger powder (1 to 2 grams) along with water.
- Take approx. 10 to 20 g of soda bicarbonate and mix with 250 ml warm water. Use this mixture as a local application on the affected skin.
- Pound some raw turmeric and take ½ to 1 tsp of the powder mixed in a glass of warm milk once or twice daily.

ECZEMA
Ayurvedic Name *Vicharchika*

Characteristic Symptoms
- Extremely itchy and erythematic papules or small vesicles, which start from the cheeks and spread to the other parts of the body.
- The vesicles rupture and the fluid oozes out leaving behind crusts which further dry out and residual pigmentation remains.

Ayurvedic View
Eczema is believed to be a minor type of leprosy caused mainly by an aggravation of the *kapha dosha* along with vitiation of the other two body humors, the *vatta* and *pitta doshas*.

Management by Home Cures
- Apply the juice of wheat grass to the affected skin and also drink approx. 50 ml twice a day. It acts as a natural antiseptic.
- Boil some coconut oil with a few cloves of garlic. Filter it, then allow it to cool down gradually; apply on the affected skin 2 or 3 times daily.
- Wash the area with a decoction prepared by boiling a few leaves of *neem*.
- Pound mustard seeds to make a paste. Cut and fill the stem of *snuhi* with this paste; cover with clay and cook. Remove from the fire and allow it to cool down

gradually. Mix it in mustard oil and apply locally at the site of the skin infection.
- Mix coconut oil with some camphor. Apply it on the affected skin.
- Wash the area with a decoction prepared by boiling the powder of the three *myrobalans* (*aamla, harad* and *baheda*).
- Take 2 or 3 juvenile leaves of *neem*. Pound them along with 2 or 3 black peppercorns and make into small balls. Take 1 or 2 balls on an empty stomach twice.
- Apply turmeric paste locally or take approx. ½ tsp twice with milk.

LEUCODERMA
Ayurvedic Name   Shwitra, Kilas

Characteristic Symptoms
- Patches of de-pigmentation of the skin, generally surrounded by skin with increased pigmentation.
- Appearance of white-coloured hair in the macules.
- As the malady proceeds the patches might spread extensively covering the entire skin surface.

Ayurvedic View
According to Ayurveda, leucoderma is caused by morbidity of the liver, which results in deficiency of the *pitta* or fire body humor. Vitiation of the body humors later involves the *rakta* (blood), *mansa* (flesh) and *medha* (fat) tissues, which result in the formation of white patches on the skin.

Management by Home Cures
- Pound the seeds of *bakuchi*, along with water, to make a paste. Apply this paste to the affected skin.
- Mix 1 to 3 g of the powder of *bakuchi* seeds with honey. Take it twice a day.
- Pound a few leaves of holy basil to extract the juice. Apply on the patches 2 or 3 times daily.
- Take 3 to 5 juvenile leaves of *neem* on an empty stomach in the morning.
- Pound the roots of *chitrak* to prepare a paste. Apply on the affected areas.

- It is important to keep the bowels moving. Take 3 to 5 g of *trifla* powder at night along with warm water or milk.
- Mix together the oils extracted from *bakuchi*, *neem*, sandalwood and *chalmogra*. Apply on the patches twice a day. For best results apply the oil and expose the skin patches to direct sunlight for about ten minutes.
- Pound basil to extract the juice. Massage it on the white patches.

ACNE
Ayurvedic Name *Yuvan Pidika*

Characteristic Symptoms
- This is found more often in adolescents when there is excessive secretion from the oil glands. It tends to disappear with age.
- Presence of open or closed comedomes.
- Presence of pus-filled pustules, inflamed papules or nodules. The cysts leave scars on erupting.

Ayurvedic View
Distortion in the air and phlegm humors causes further distortion of the blood or *rakta dhatu*.

Management by Home Cures
- Prepare a paste by adding some water to cinnamon powder. Apply on the affected area, acne or boils, for relief from inflammation as well as pain.
- Coconut oil contains anti-microbial and antiseptic properties. This is why the external use of coconut oil is considered beneficial in curing acne.
- Pound the seeds of *chironji, masoor* and *sarson* to prepare a paste. Apply the paste to the pustules.
- Make a paste by grinding nutmeg and apply on acne.
- Apply curd (yoghurt) on the affected skin locally.
- Roast some orange lentils (*masoor dal*) in ghee. Allow to cool down gradually. Make a paste with milk and apply

on the pimples. Allow it to dry, then gently remove with cold water.

- Pound raw turmeric and take 3 to 5 g of the powder along with water or mixed into honey twice a day.
- Dry some orange peel in the shade and make into a powder. Apply this, mixed in a little raw milk, on the affected skin.
- Prepare a paste by pounding *kali mirch*, *lal chandan* and *jaiphal* and apply locally.
- Apply the juice of wheat grass on the affected skin and also drink 100 ml per day. It acts as a blood purifier and is a natural antiseptic.
- Steam the face while boiling a few leaves of basil and *neem* in water. Pat dry with a clean towel afterwards.
- Local application as well as intake of coconut water helps.
- For getting rid of the pimples or boils, take some black pepper powder and add a little ghee to it. Apply on the affected area.
- Take 2 tsp rose syrup mixed in a glassful of water on an empty stomach once or twice a day to cure heat-induced skin ailments like pimples. Apply rose water externally to the skin.

BOILS
Ayurvedic Name *Vidradhi*

Characteristic Symptoms
- One or more papules on the exposed parts of the body.
- The papules may be dry or ulcerative, covered with crust and oozing a sticky secretion.

Ayurvedic View
This disease is believed to be caused by the vitiation in the body humors, *vatta*, *pitta* and *kapha*, or an imbalance of all the three *doshas*.

Management by Home Cures
- Wash the boils with a decoction prepared by boiling *neem* leaves.
- The powder of the 3 *myrobalans* can be boiled and used to wash the boils.
- Soak a few almonds in water, then remove the skins; pound them along with a few *neem* leaves and some black peppercorns. Form into small balls. Take 1 or 2, twice a day, with warm water. This works as a blood purifier.
- Mix some black pepper powder and a little ghee together and apply on the affected areas.
- A poultice of powdered *methi* seeds and turmeric powder can be tied twice a day.
- Mix the powder of catechu in water to make a paste. Use

as a local application. It has the benefit of an antiseptic and anti-pruritic drug.
- Semi-baked onion can be applied on the boil. This would help to ripen and then open and drain the boil.
- Mix cinnamon powder with some water to make a paste. Apply this paste over the affected area for relief from inflammation as well as pain.
- Pound the seeds of *methi* to make a paste. Warm this and apply on the site of the boil.
- Prepare a powder of equal parts of fennel and dry coriander; add double the quantity of powdered *mishri*: Take approx. 3 to 5 g of this powder twice daily for some days. For children the dose would be half.
- Apply the juice of wheat grass on the affected skin. It acts as a blood purifier and natural antiseptic. You could also take 50 ml of the juice twice a day.

HAIR LOSS
Ayurvedic Name *Khalitya*

Characteristic Symptoms
- Temporary or permanent loss of hair from the scalp.
- May be due to hereditary, emotional or malnutritional factors.
- Sometimes it remains irreversible.

Ayurvedic View
The *pitta* humor that is present in the distal end of the pores of the hair is affected by distortion in the air body humor. This causes falling hair.

Management by Home Cures
- Mix some lemon juice in double the quantity of coconut oil. Use this mixture to massage the scalp and leave it on for about half an hour before washing the hair.
- Wash the hair on alternate days or twice a week with a decoction of *mulathi*.
- Massage the scalp and hair with oil of *bhringraj*.
- Pound a few fresh leaves of kareer and make into a paste with water. Apply on the scalp.
- Pound the seeds of *kalaunji* to make a paste. Apply locally at the site of the hair loss.
- A thorough massage of the scalp performed daily with the fingertips improves the blood circulation and thereby prevents hair fall.

- Pound garlic cloves along with a pinch of callyrium; mix in butter and apply the paste on the affected skin.
- Pound *kadva parval* to extract the juice. Use this juice for local massage on the scalp.
- Pound mango kernels and mix the powder in *aamla* juice. Apply this mixture on the scalp and give a gentle massage before a bath.
- Mix the powder of dried *aamla* with honey. Take it twice a day. Washing the hair with aamla powder helps.
- Apply a paste of carrot on the scalp. Leave it on for 15-20 minutes and wash thoroughly. Repeat for some days.
- Add henna leaves to some mustard oil and heat together on low heat to make a medicated hair oil at home.
- Pound the flowers of hibiscus to make a paste; mix into cow's urine. Apply on the scalp.
- Pound fresh coriander to extract the juice. Massage lightly on the scalp.
- An easy cure for hair ailments like premature greying and loss of hair is to massage the scalp with sesame oil which encourages hair growth.
- Take 1 tsp of a powdered mixture of the herbs *aamla*, *harad* and *baheda* preferably with lukewarm water once or twice daily for some days.
- Apply some juice of wheat grass to your scalp to combat dandruff and loss of hair. Take a bath with water containing a few drops of wheat grass. This works as a natural cleanser.

OSTEOARTHRITIS

Ayurvedic Name *Sandhigat Vaata*

Characteristic Symptoms

- Tenderness and enlargement of the joint with limitation in its movements.
- Pain in the affected joints, which increases on movement and decreases with rest.
- Articular stiffness and wasting of the muscles.
- The pain might increase with change in the weather.

Ayurvedic View

This disease is believed to result from vitiation of the *vatta* dosha. The vitiated *vatta* present in the joints tends to cause deformity or dislocation of the joint, pain and swelling.

Management by Home Cures

- Warm mustard oil or sesame oil and mix with powdered dried ginger. Massage into the joint.
- Being slimy and hot, groundnuts cause a decrease in the *vatta* or the air body humor. A local massage of warmed groundnut oil is recommended.
- A massage of mustard oil provides strength and warmth to the joints and muscles of the body and relieves pain. It acts as a rubefacient
  (refers to external application that causes redness of the skin) that relieves muscular pain and stiffness.

- Warm some sesame oil or mustard oil and mix the powders of turmeric, garlic and camphor into it. This is an effective massage oil for joint pains.
- The seeds and leaves of papaya will decrease pain and swelling. In the case of joint pains, warm the leaves and apply as a hot fomentation onto the affected joints; or; the seeds can be crushed and mixed into mustard oil for local massage.
- Add camphor to mustard oil, sesame oil or any medicated oil. Use locally to relieve inflammation, swelling as well as pain.
- Sesame helps to subside the *vatta dosha* or air body humor which, when aggravated, causes muscle and joint pains. Soak some black sesame seeds in a glass of water overnight. Drink this water along with the seeds in the morning.

RHEUMATOID ARTHRITIS
Ayurvedic Name   *Aamvaata*

Characteristic Symptoms
- Generally polyarthritis, with pain, stiffness and symmetrical swelling of the peripheral joints.
- The small joints of the fingers and toes are affected first.
- Morning stiffness.
- Skin may develop subcutaneous fibrous nodules.
- Anorexia, weakness, loss of weight and characteristic deformities of the joints as the disease progresses.
- The R. A. factor is positive.

Ayurvedic View
Weakness of the gastric fire causes food to remain undigested. The undigested juice or the endotoxins, *aam rasa*, intermingle with the vitiated humor of *vatta*. This causes pain and inflammation in the joints.

Management by Home Cures
- Mix a pinch of saffron in a glass of warmed cow's milk. Take it at bedtime.
- Mix 5 to 10 ml purified *erand* oil in milk or water. Take it at bedtime.
- Add camphor to mustard oil, sesame oil or any medicated oil. Massage locally to relieve the inflammation as well as pain.
- Warm some clove oil and massage it into the site of the pain.

- Mix dried ginger powder into sesame oil and massage into the joint. Take approx. 3 g dried ginger powder twice daily along with warm water.
- A local massage of warmed groundnut oil is recommended.
- A local massage of warmed mustard oil is recommended.
- Heat a bag of sand and use as a hot compress over the painful and swollen joint.
- Heat the leaves of *dhatura*, then use them as a hot compress or tie to the affected joint as a poultice.
- Prepare a decoction by boiling *rasna* and *giloy* in equal parts. Add ¼ tsp dried ginger powder. Take approx. 20 ml, lukewarm, twice daily.
- Warm the leaves of papaya and apply as a hot fomentation on the affected joints; or crush the seeds and mix into mustard oil for local massage.
- Sesame helps to reduce the *vatta dosha* or air body humor and provides relief.
- Prepare a decoction by boiling *amarbel*. Use this as a hot fomentation.
- Fry small pieces of ginger in ghee made from cow's milk. Take a few of these with daily meals.

GOUT
Ayurvedic Name *Vaata Rakta*

Characteristic Symptoms
- Throbbing pain that starts from a single joint and later spreads to other joints.
- The joints are hot, painful and swollen with shiny skin.
- There may be disability and deformity of the joints in chronic cases.
- Loss of function and movement as the disease progresses.
- Serum uric acid gets elevated.

Ayurvedic View
This disease is caused by the vitiation of the *vatta* or the air body humor. An improper diet and improper elimination of metabolic wastes from the body are the predisposing factors.

Management by Home Cures
- Take 2 to 4 cloves of garlic on an empty stomach.
- Take a decoction of approx. 50 ml *manjishtha* twice a day.
- Fry small pieces of ginger in ghee made from cow's milk. Take a few of these with daily meals.
- Mix powdered dried ginger into sesame oil and massage into the joint.
- Boil the root bark of the *ashvattha* tree. Take approx. 50 ml of this decoction twice a day.

- Pound the dried fruit of harad to make a powder. Take 3 to 5 g along with warm water once or twice a day.
- Soak a few seeds of *methi* in a glass of water overnight. In the morning mash and mix with 1 tsp honey.
- Pound some *methi* seeds and some dried ginger. Mix 1 tsp of each powder into some jaggery and take this twice daily.

LUMBAR SPONDYLITIS
Ayurvedic Name *Teevar Prishtha Shoola*

Characteristic Symptoms
- Pain and stiffness in the back that is more during the mornings.
- Restriction of the lumbar spine movements.
- Pain is more on the sacro-iliac compression.
- Osteoporosis may be an accompanying feature.

Ayurvedic View
Distortion or vitiation in the body humors causes this disease. An aggravation in the *vatta* humor is the predisposing cause.

Management by Home Cures
- Mix 1 tsp powdered raw turmeric and ¼ tsp dried ginger powder in a glass of warm milk and take it at bedtime.
- Roast and powder *methi* seeds and take approx. 3 to 5 g along with hot milk or water twice a day.
- Prepare a decoction of dried ginger and some pure castor oil. Take approx ½ cup, warmed, at bedtime.
- Dissolve some camphor in mustard oil and warm it till it is tolerably hot. Massage into the site of the pain.

EPILEPSY

Ayurvedic Name   *Apasmaar*

Characteristic Symptoms

- In Grand mal there is a dreamy stage when there are mood changes, irritability, depression, euphoria and tension. Sudden jerks in the limbs; a feeling of choking; sudden loss of consciousness; powerful jerking movements of the face, limbs and body. Urine may be passed involuntarily; frothy saliva in the mouth; afterwards the movements cease and consciousness is regained; headache; fatigue and confusion.
- In petit mal there is a temporary loss of consciousness, but the patient regains consciousness faster.
- In partial epilepsy, there are emotional changes, hallucinations, irrelevant behaviour and talk.
- In status epilepticus, there are continuous fits without any recovery.

Ayurvedic View

Apasmaar is caused by vitiation in either of the 3 humors, air, heat and phlegm, or from a combined disharmony in all 3 humors. There are 4 types:

a. Caused by vitiation in the *vatta* or the air body humor.
b. Caused by distortion of *pitta* or the heat.
c. Caused by vitiation in the *kapha* or phlegm.
d. Caused by vitiation in all the 3 humors of the body.

Management by Home Cures

- Massage sesame oil into the scalp and also on the soles of the feet.
- Increase the intake of almonds in the diet.
- Pound the roots of *vacha* into a powder and take approx. 1 tsp with milk twice daily.
- Take the powder of *shatavari* along with the powder or juice of *bramhi* twice.
- Crush the fruit of *aamla* and take 30 ml of the fresh juice on an empty stomach.
- Extract the juice by pounding a few cloves of garlic. Put this as ear drops.
- Deeply inhale ghee made from cow's milk through both the nostrils twice daily.

GIDDINESS
Ayurvedic Name   *Bhram Roga*

Characteristic Symptoms
- A strange feeling that the external environment is spinning.
- There may be a sensation of moving objects around the patient. A sudden or severe movement might make him fall down.

Ayurvedic View
When *raja guna* increases beyond its normal limits, it causes an imbalance in the air and fire body humors. This causes a disruption in the balance in the brain, resulting in vertigo.

Management by Home Cures
- Pound the roots of *ashwagandha* to make a powder. Take 1 tsp along with warm milk twice a day.
- Pound approx. 1 large tsp dry coriander seeds. Remove the husk and boil the seeds in a glassful of milk; add some sugar and take it preferably at bedtime.
- Pound *malkangni* into a powder. Take approx. 1 to 2 g twice for a few days.
- Local massage of the scalp with oil of *aamla* and *bramhi* is recommended.
- Soak 20 g *moong* dal in water overnight. In the morning remove the outer skin and pound the dal. To this add approx. 10 g ghee and boil the mixture in 250 ml milk for

some time; remove from fire and add sugar. Take this twice a day.
- Pound approx. 50 g of dried *shankhpushpi*. To this add an equal amount of powdered *mishri*. Take 1 to 2 tsp of this mixture once or twice daily preferably with warmed cow's milk.

SLEEPLESSNESS
Ayurvedic Name *Anidra*

Characteristic Symptoms
- Loss or disturbance in the pattern of sleep.
- Insufficient depth or duration of sleep, generally causing early awakening.

Ayurvedic View
Any vitiation in one or more of the 3 body humors - air, heat or phlegm, along with an increase in the *rajas guna*, causes this disease. Sometimes a distortion in all the 3 *doshas* tends to cause loss of sleep.

Management by Home Cures
- Pound the dried roots of *ashwagandha* to make a powder. Take 3 to 5 g at bedtime with warm and sweetened milk.
- Prepare a decoction by boiling mint leaves. Allow to cool down gradually. Take the decoction slightly warmed with 1 tsp powdered *mishri* or honey. Repeat it at bedtime for some days.
- Fry approx. 1 tsp powdered cumin seeds in *desi* ghee and pound them. Mix them into the pulp of a ripe banana. Take this at bedtime.
- A local massage of almond oil on the scalp and also taking a few drops of the almond oil mixed in sweetened, buffalo's hot milk at bedtime is recommended.

- Immerse the feet in warm water for ten minutes and thereafter massage the soles with mustard oil. Try this practice daily for a few days before going to bed.
- Take approx. 125 to 250 mg *hing* powder twice a day in the form of a condiment.
- If you occasionally suffer from sleeplessness, try this home remedy: Pound approx. 1 large tsp dry coriander seeds; remove the husk and boil the seeds in a glassful of milk. Take this warm with some sugar preferably at bedtime.
- Increase the intake of raw white onions in salad.
- Henna is also effective in the treatment of sleep disorders. Prepare a decoction out of the flowers of henna; cool and add sugar. Take approx. ¼ cup at bedtime. To complement the results, you could spread some fresh henna flowers on your pillow. The sweet and soothing fragrance will ensure a good night's sleep.
- Increase the intake of papaya if you remain sleepless occasionally.

SCIATICA
Ayurvedic Name *Gridhrasi*

Characteristic Symptoms
- Pain travels in the region of the sciatic nerve. It starts from the buttock and radiates down in the posterior aspect of the thigh and calf and in the outer border of the foot.
- Numbness and a tingling sensation may be felt in the region of the affected nerve.
- Restriction of movement and pain while raising the straightened leg.

Ayurvedic View
Sciatica or *gridhrasi* is caused by vitiation in the *vatta* and *kapha doshas* or the air and phlegm body humors. Constipation and physical strain aggravate the disease.

Management by Home Cures
- Mix saffron in warm milk and take it once or twice, preferably at bedtime.
- Take 1 or 2 tsp purified castor oil mixed in milk preferably at bedtime.
- Take approx. 125 to 500 mg *hing*.
- Heat a bag of salt and use it as a hot fomentation on the affected leg.
- Swallow 2 to 4 cloves of garlic along with water on an empty stomach in the morning.

- Mix 1 g each of dried ginger powder and *pippali* powder, and 5 to 10 ml of castor oil. Take this mixture once or twice daily for a few days.
- Dry the leaves of *harsingar* in the shade and pound into a powder. Take approx. 3 g mixed with honey twice a day.
- Massage warm clove oil into the site of the pain.

ANXIETY
Ayurvedic Name *Chhitodveg*

Characteristic Symptoms
A variety of symptoms may be present:
- Loss of sleep; disturbed sleep
- Loss of appetite
- Mental instability and depression
- Occasional pain in the chest; palpitations; excessive perspiration; giddiness; loss of breath and fainting

Ayurvedic View
The main cause of this disease is the imbalance in the normal values of the mind with increase in the *rajas* and *tamas* states. These may also cause a distortion in the body humors.

Management by Home Cures
- Put the freshly extracted juice of basil leaves in the nostrils as nasal drops. Basil soothes the brain, relieves anxiety, boosts intellect and acts as a nerve tonic.
- Pound dried *shankhpushpi* into a powder. Take 1 tsp twice daily along with warm cow's milk.
- Use ghee made from cow's milk, or almond oil as nasal drops 2 or 3 times a day.
- Increase the use of *petha* (white gourd) in your regular meals. Crush the pulp of *petha* and extract the fresh juice. Take 10 to 20 ml twice a day.
- Pound *bramhi* to extract the juice. Take approx. 20 ml twice or thrice.

URINARY TRACT INFECTION
Ayurvedic Name *Mootrakrichha*

Characteristic Symptoms
- Fever along with shivering, pain and burning while passing urine and increased frequency of urination
- An aching pain in the loins and flanks
- A persistent desire to urinate even though the bladder is empty.
- Laboratory findings show increased pus cells in the urine.

Ayurvedic View
This ailment is believed to be a manifestation of vitiation in any of the body humors or all 3 humors - air, fire and phlegm. An aggravation of *pitta* is the predominant cause.

Management by Home Cures
- Grate cucumber to extract the juice. Take approx. 20 to 30 ml, 2 or 3 times.
- Soak approx. 10 g seeds of coriander in water overnight. In the morning pound them into a drink, strain and take it mixed with 1 tsp *mishri*.
- Pound a piece of cinnamon into a powder. Take 1 to 3 along with a glassful of water.
- Take coconut water 3 to 4 times a day.
- Mix approx. 10 g of pure *shilajit* powder, 100 g powdered seeds of *jamun* and 100 g of powdered *Shimla ke mool* (Baricum root). Take about 3 to 5 g of this mixture on an empty stomach.

- Mix 2 tsp of the freshly extracted juice of green *amlas* and about 1 small tsp honey in ½ glass lukewarm water. Take at least twice a day.
- Grapes are also a natural diuretic. In case of urinary disorders try to increase the intake of grapes.
- Prepare a decoction by boiling the roots and stem of *punarnava*. Take approx. 20 ml twice a day.
- Sandalwood contains anti-infective and anti-bacterial properties which decrease the pus cells in the urine. Boil approx. 3 to 5 g of the flakes or powder of sandalwood to prepare a decoction. Dissolve some sugar or *mishri* in it and take 3 or 4 times.
- Pound fresh coriander leaves to extract their juice. Mix a spoon of powdered *mishri* to 10 to 15 ml juice and take twice.

URINARY RETENTION
Ayurvedic Name *Mootrkshaya*

Characteristic Symptoms
- Poor force of urine with pain, in the form of dribbling or a thin stream.
- The urinary bladder is distended and tender to touch.
- The urine volume is reduced to less than 400 ml in 24 hours.
- The urge to urinate persists even after urination.

Ayurvedic View
According to *Ayurvedic* texts, there are eight forms of the disease. Three types are caused by the vitiation of the *vatta, pitta* and *kapha doshas*, or the air, heat and phlegm body humors. The fourth type is a result of an imbalance in all the three *doshas*. The fifth one is due to the failure of the system to expel wastes. The remaining two types are due to the presence of stones in the bladder.

Management by Home Cures
- Boil the root of *pashanabheda* to prepare a decoction. Take approx. 50 ml twice a day.
- Prepare a mixture of approx. 1 g powder of *yavkshara* and 5 g powder of the fruit of *gokhru*. Take this with water twice a day.
- Take 20 to 30 ml decoction of the bark of the *varuna* tree 2 or 3 times.
- Take approx. 1 g cardamom powder along with water or milk once or twice a day.

- Mix together 1 g of the powder of *kalmishora* and 1 g of the powder of *yavkshar*. Take it along with water twice a day.
- Crush radish along with its leaves to extract the juice. Take approx. 20 ml twice daily.
- Camphor gives a natural stimulus to the kidneys, causing a free flow of the urine. Take 125 to 375 mg camphor either mixed in sweetened milk or with sugar.
- Pound a piece of cinnamon bark to make a powder. Take 1 to 3 g along with a glassful of water.
- Fresh coconut water is diuretic and is recommended.
- Boil a few leaves of mint to prepare a decoction; let it cool then add some *mishri* or sugar. Take 20 to 40 ml every 4 hours.
- Boil approx. 3 to 5 g of the flakes or powder of sandalwood to prepare a decoction and dissolve some sugar or *mishri* in it. Take this 3 or 4 times.

URINARY STONES
Ayurvedic Name *Mootrashmari*

Characteristic Symptoms
- Supra pubic or renal pain which is normally first intermittent and dull in nature, and later on manifests in the region of the loin or back.
- The pain generally increases on movement.
- A continuous urge to pass urine; many cases show interruption and frequency in the flow of urine.
- Sometimes expulsion of blood with the urine.
- Other visible symptoms are fever, loss of appetite, nausea and vomiting, and painful urination.
- X-ray of the urinary tract would suggest the position, size and shape of the stone. A radio opaque shadow is visible.

Ayurvedic View
The 4 types of *ashmari* are:
1. Caused by vitiation of *vatta* or air body humor
2. Caused by vitiation of *pitta* or fire body humor
3. Caused by vitiation of *kapha* or phlegm body humor
4. Formed from dried semen

Management by Home Cures
- Take 1 g *shilajit* twice a day.
- Take 1 tsp of the powdered rhizome of *pashanbheda* 2 to 3 times along with a glassful of water.
- Take 1 g of the powder of *yavkshara* 3 times with water.

- Prepare a decoction by boiling the bark of the varuna tree. Take approx. 30 ml of the decoction 2 or 3 times a day.
- Take a radish and hollow it out. Fill it with a mixture of approx. 2 g carrot seeds and 2 grams turnip seeds. Heat it on a charcoal fire till it turns into ashes. When the radish has been roasted, remove the seed mixture and take 3 to 6 g along with water for a few days.
- Make a decoction of *kulthi* seeds. Take in a dose of 30 ml twice a day.
- Take 3 to 5 g of the powder of *harad* with *mishri* to relieve the problems of decreased urination and help to flush out small stones of the urinary tract.
- Take the powder of gum *guggul* in a dose of 2 to 4 g twice daily for some days. This is helpful in breaking down urinary stones.
- Soak approx. 50 g of the pulse *kulthi* in water overnight. In the morning mash it and drink it.

BLOOD IN URINE

Ayurvedic Name *Raktameha, Adhoga Rakta Pitta*

Characteristic Symptoms

- Presence of blood in the urine, which causes the colour of urine to be red, reddish-brown or smoky.
- Bleeding may occur while passing urine or in the form of a few drops afterwards.
- Pain in the loins may be present.
- Normally, the colour of the urine is bright red when the stone, while moving inside the urethra, tends to scratch it. On the other hand, if it is present in the kidneys or the bladder, then the urine shows a brownish hue.
- If the blood appears before the urine, it is most likely that the reason lies in the bladder; and if the urine contains blood, then chances are that any part of the urinary tract other than the urethra is the cause.

Ayurvedic View

According to Ayurveda, this disease is a variety of *adhog raktapitta*. This is specified by the downward vitiation of the *pitta* body humor in blood.

Management by Home Cures

- Take approx. 1 g of the powder of *shilajit* along with lukewarm milk twice a day.
- Take approx. 1 tsp of the powdered seeds of *gokshur* with honey and milk.
- Extract the juice of raw *karela* by crushing it. Take approx. 20 ml twice a day.

- Take ½ to 1 tsp of the juice of fresh leaves of *vasa* 3 or 4 times a day.
- Crush *petha* to extract the juice. Take 20 to 30 ml twice a day.

RENAL COLIC
Ayurvedic Name *Vrukk Shool*

Characteristic Symptoms
- The most important symptom of renal colic is pain due to the presence of stones which cause irritation or a blockage.
- The pain is normally dull and intermittent; it radiates from the loins to the genitals.
- During the bouts of intense pain, the patient rolls on his abdomen and nothing seems to provide relief.
- Other symptoms are nausea, vomiting and intense perspiration.
- Sometimes there is a continuous urge to urinate although the bladder is empty.

Ayurvedic View
An aggravation or vitiation of the *vatta dosha* or body humor is the predominant cause of colicky renal pain.

Management by Home Cures
- Take approx. 20 ml of a decoction of *kulthi* twice or thrice.
- Boil the roots of *erand* and *yavkshar* to make a decoction. Take approx. 30 ml twice.
- Make a powder by mixing the following ingredients: *kala jeera*, *ajwain* and *kala namak* in the ratio of 4:2:1. Take approx. 3 to 5 g of the powder 3 or 4 times with warm water.
- Take 1 g *shilajit* 2 or 3 times with water.

PROSTATE ENLARGEMENT
Ayurvedic Name *Ashtheela*

Characteristic Symptoms
- The enlargement of the prostate gland causes an obstruction in the normal exit of urine from the bladder.
- An increased frequency and urgency in passing urine; there may also be pain during urination.
- The patient tends to pass urine many times at night and in many cases there is a feelingof burning along with the passage of urine.
- A persistent pain in the genitals and the lower back.
- Recurrent urinary tract infection; blood may be present in urine in advanced stages.
- On rectal examination, the prostate gland is enlarged and tender to touch. On examining the abdomen the bladder is generally found to be distended.

Ayurvedic View
This disease is believed to develop from vitiation in one of the 3 body humors, *vatta*, *pitta* and *kapha*. Or it may be a consequence of the distortion of all the 3 *doshas*.

Management by Home Cures
- Prepare a mixture of powdered cucumber seeds and black salt in the ratio of 20:1. Take approx. 250 ml with *kanji* (fermented drink prepared from black carrots) twice daily for relief.
- Take 1 g *shilajit* twice with warm milk.

- Take 50 ml of the juice of fresh *petha* and add 1 g of *yavkshara*. Take this 2 or 3 times with some sugar.
- Prepare a decoction from the roots of *erand* and *yavkshar*. Take approx. 30 ml twice.
- Take approx. 10 to 20 ml purified castor oil mixed in water or milk, twice.
- Soak 2 or 3 dried *anjeer* in water overnight. In the morning mash the *anjeer* and drink the mixture. Continue for a few days.
- Dip a small woollen blanket in a cow's warm urine. Foment the bladder with this for relief.
- Prepare a mixture by pounding together equal quantities (approx. 3 g) of cumin seeds and *mishri*. Take this with water twice a day.

BED WETTING

Characteristic Symptoms
- Involuntary passing of urine usually during sleep at night.
- The reason may be physical or even emotional. Organic defects in the urinary tract; any infection or even the presence of worms.
- More commonly found in young children.

Ayurvedic View
Vitiation in either or all the humors, viz. air, fire and phlegm, causes this malady.

Management by Home Cures
- Take approx 20 ml of the fresh juice of *amla* on an empty stomach.
- Make the child lick some salt just before going to bed.
- Take a glassful of warm milk with a pinch or two of saffron.
- Prepare a decoction by boiling approx. 20 g of *vidanga*. Take twice with ½ tsp honey. This helps to cure the problem of bedwetting and also helps to destroy intestinal worms.
- Roast 1 tsp black sesame seeds along with double the amount of jaggery. Take it warm along with warm milk once or twice a day.
- Take approx. 50 g of black sesame seeds and half the quantity of *ajwain*. Roast the seeds and add an equal

quantity of jaggery to the mixture. Take this twice a day along with warm milk.
- Make the child eat a tsp of dried grapes and the kernel of a walnut for some days before going to bed at night.
- Give the child 1 tsp honey at bedtime.
- Take ¼ to ½ g purified *shilajit* powder twice a day along with warm cow's milk.

LEUCORRHOEA

Ayurvedic Name *Shwetpradra*

Characteristic Symptoms
- Varied types of discharge from the vagina.
- Discharge may be colourless, whitish or yellowish to greenish.
- There may or may not be a foul smell.
- Itching, discomfort, general weakness, vaginitis and dyspareunia (painful intercourse) may be present.

Ayurvedic View
According to Ayurvedic texts, leucorrhoea is caused by a vitiation of *kapha* or the phlegm body humor.

Management by Home Cures
- Take approx. 20 to 30 ml of an infusion prepared by boiling and cooling freshly pounded coriander, twice.
- Prepare a decoction by boiling the bark of the banyan tree. Use this as a vaginal douche.
- The liquid extract from the bark of the mango tree can be used to cure leucorrhoea.
- Take 1 tsp powdered *mulethi* and add double the quantity of ground *mishri*. Take this twice with water for a few days.
- Take approx. 50 ml rice water 2 or 3 times for a few days.
- Pound the fresh roots of asparagus. Take 3 to 6 g mixed with milk once or twice, preferably on an empty stomach.

- Mix equal parts of powdered *karkat shringi* and *majuphala*. Take approx. 3 g of this mixture along with water twice a day.
- Grind a few leaves of *sheesham* in water. Strain and take approx. 20 to 30 ml of this juice twice for a few days.
- Take approx. 3 to 5 g *amla* powder twice a day mixed in 1 tsp honey.
- Wash the vaginal area regularly with *phitkari* dissolved in water.
- Take some rose petals and grind them into a paste; add *mishri* or honey. Take this twice along with lukewarm milk.
- Washing the vaginal area with a decoction prepared by boiling *neem* leaves could be of help.
- Take a glassful of carrot juice mixed with ½ tsp honey for a few days.

PAINFUL MENSTRUATION
Ayurvedic Name *Kashatartav*

Characteristic Symptoms
- Colicky, cramping pain in the lower abdomen along with or before the onset of the menstrual cycle.
- A constant dull ache which is usually relieved with menstruation.
- Nausea, fatigue, abdominal distention, irritability, and frequency in urination and sometimes diarrhoea.
- The symptoms of primary dysmenorrhoea (painful menses) disappear with age in many cases.

Ayurvedic View
Vitiation of the 3 humors, *vatta, pitta* and *kapha* causes this ailment. More particularly it is the aggravation of the *vatta dosha* that is the predisposing cause of painful menses.

Management by Home Cures
- Mix ½ to 1 g saffron in warm milk and take at bedtime.
- Women who suffer from painful menstrual flow should increase their intake of garlic during menses.
- Take 20 to 30 ml of the juice extracted by crushing the raw fruit of pineapple twice a day.
- Regular intake of raw onions is also beneficial in relieving abdominal cramps. Take 10 to 30 ml onion juice twice a day.
- Roast 1 or 2 tsp sesame seeds and mix into some

jaggery. Heat on low flame and take it warm once or twice a day.
- Pound *kalaunji* seeds into a powder: Take 1 to 3 g twice along with warm water.
- Hot fomentation of the lower part of the abdomen is indeed relieving.

EXCESSIVE MENSTRUATION
Ayurvedic Name *Rakta Pradar*

Characteristic Symptoms
- Excessive bleeding during the menstrual cycle.
- Sometimes the menses last for a prolonged duration. Anaemia might follow.

Ayurvedic View
The disease is believed to be the result of the imbalance of hormones caused by a distortion in the heat or *pitta* body humor.

Management by Home Cures
- Crush red *punarnava* to extract the juice. Take 5 to 10 ml. twice daily.
- An enema prepared by adding *phitkari* to water in the ratio of 1:5 is recommended.
- Crush the fruit of *amla* and extract the juice. Take approx. 20 ml, preferably on an empty stomach.
- Mix some *phitkari* powder in water and use it as a vaginal wash.
- Pound 7 tender leaves of pomegranate and 7 grains of rice to form a paste. Take this twice daily for a few days.
- Use the liquid extracted from the bark of the mango tree to cure heavy bleeding.
- Approx. ½ tsp *phitkari* powder can also be taken twice mixed in milk.
- Pound the juvenile flowers of hibiscus into a paste along with some milk. Take 5 to 10 g of the paste 2 times a day.

SCANTY MENSTRUATION
Ayurvedic Name *Anartava, Nashtartava*

Characteristic Symptoms
* Absence of menstruation, even after the age of menarche.
* Decreased or very little amount of bleeding during the menses.
* Sometimes, secondary amenorrhoea (lack of menstruation) in which there is absence of menses for a long period in a woman who earlier had menstruation.

Ayurvedic View
Vitiation of the body humors is believed to be the cause of this disease.

Management by Home Cures
* Pound equal quantities of dried ginger, *ajwain*, black sesame seeds and jaggery to make a powder. Take 3 to 6 g twice a day along with warm water.
* Boil carrot seeds to make a decoction. Take 15 to 30 ml twice.
* Pound the dried seeds of carrots and radishes. Take 1 g of the powder twice with warm water.
* Saffron has also been successfully used for treating womens' ailments like scanty menses and amenorrhoea. A pinch or two can be taken mixed in a glassful of warm milk.

- Boil the powders of soya and *kalaunji* and the root bark of the cotton plant to make a decoction. Add jaggery and take approx. 50 ml, warmed, twice a day.
- Women suffering from scanty menses should increase their intake of garlic and raw onions.
- Pound some sesame seeds and mix with jaggery. Take approx 20 g twice.
- Extract fresh juice from aloe vera. Take 20 to 30 ml two times.
- Crush the raw fruit of pineapple and extract the juice. Take 20 to 30 ml twice a day.

DIFFERENTIAL UTERINE BLEEDING
Ayurvedic Name   *Rakta Pradar*

Characteristic Symptoms
- Painless, irregular and heavy bleeding generally in the form of clots.
- There may be a period of amenorrhoea, oligomenorrhoea and inter-menstrual spotting.

Ayurvedic View
This ailment results from change in the hormone levels due to an aggravation or distortion in the normal working of *pitta* or the heat humor of the body.

Management by Home Cures
- Wash the effected area regularly with *phitkari* mixed with water. An enema prepared with *phitkari* and water in the ratio of 1:5 is recommended.
- Take equal quantities of powdered *naagkesar*, *lodhra* and *mochras* and mix them. Take approx. 1 g of the mixture twice a day along with rice water.
- Pound the juvenile flowers of hibiscus along with some milk to make a paste. Take 5 to 10 g of the paste twice a day.
- Pound the dried pollen of *nagkeshar*. Take approx. 1 to 3 g of the powder along with milk or water twice a day.
- Take approx. ½ tsp *phitkari* powder twice, mixed in milk.
- Crush red *punarnava* to extract the juice. Take 5 to 10 ml twice daily.

GOITRE
Ayurvedic Name *Galaganda*

Characteristic Symptoms
- Swelling in the neck without any other symptoms.
- The thyroid gland may be soft, smooth and symmetrically enlarged. Multiple nodules and cysts may develop later.

Ayurvedic View
This disease results from an aggravation in the *kapha* or the phlegm and a decrease in the *pitta* or the heat body humor. This further tends to cause a distortion in the *mansa* (muscle) and *medha* (fat) *dhatus*.

Management by Home Cures
- Boil the bark of the *kachnaar* tree to prepare a decoction. Take approx. 40 to 80 ml twice a day. (1 ounce twice a day. CHANGE TO GRAMS or ML LIKE THE REST).
- Pound *jalakumbhi* to prepare a paste. Apply it over the swollen neck.
- Local application of a paste of mustard is advisable.
- Pound a few cloves of garlic and make into a paste. Tie this paste in a cloth and use as poultice over the swollen neck.
- Pound the leaves or dried roots of *ashwagandha* to make a paste. Apply over the neck.

ANAEMIA
Ayurvedic Name *Pandu Roga*

Characteristic Symptoms
- Angular stomatitis (cracks and ulcers at the angles of mouth) due to iron deficiency or anaemia.
- The nails may become flat, concave and brittle.
- There could perhaps be cardiac dilatation and an enlarged liver.

Ayurvedic View
According to Ayurveda, anaemia is caused by vitiation either in the air, fire or phlegm body humors, or imbalance in all the 3 *doshas*, or due to intake of impure mud. These vitiated *doshas* tend to affect the blood or the *rakta dhatu* causing a reduction in strength, colour and *medha dhatu*, and a decrease in the vital force.

Management by Home Cures
- Extract the juice of wheat grass. Take approx. 50 ml twice. The chlorophyll content present in wheat grass resembles (in structure as well as properties) a component of blood called haemin. It aids in improving the blood profile.
- Take 20 to 50 ml juice of pomegranate twice daily.
- Pound radish along with its leaves to extract the juice. Take 50 ml twice to build up the blood profile.
- Take ½ to 1 g of the powder of catechu with honey twice a day.

- Pound 50 g *giloy* and add some water; boil, cool and add the juice of 50 g of wheat grass. Take this mixture twice on an empty stomach.
- Pound the leaves of *neem*, mix in honey and take approx. 10 g twice.
- Extract the juice from the leaves of henna. Take 5 to 10 ml of the fresh juice twice on an empty stomach.
- Make a decoction of *punarnava*. Take approx. 20 ml, twice a day.
- Extract fresh juice from carrots, spinach and tomatoes; mix together in equal quantities. Take approx. 50 ml twice daily for a few days.
- *Jamun* tones up the liver and causes an increase in the red blood cells and improves the blood haemoglobin content.
- Take the pulp of the ripe mango regularly along with sweetened milk to increase the haemoglobin levels.
- Boil approx. 10 g cardamom seeds to prepare a decoction. Take this twice daily.

EAR DISORDERS
Ayurvedic Name *Karna Roga, Putikarna*

Characteristic Symptoms
* Pain and swelling in the lymph nodes.
* Discomfort, irritation, itching, swelling, redness and tenderness in the external ear.
* Perhaps an earache and ringing sensation in the ears.
* Perhaps loss of hearing, foul smelling discharges from the ear.
* Fever when the infection travels to the middle ear.
* Discharge of pus that may be blood stained.

Ayurvedic View
Karna Roga is caused by distortion in the body humors or from a vitiation of the *vatta* or *kapha* body humors. This initiates a pathological process that leads to ear diseases.

Management by Home Cures
* Warm onion juice and use as ear drops.
* Burn some cloves of garlic in mustard oil or coconut oil. Filter it and use as a local application.
* Boil the leaves of *nirgundi* in mustard oil; filter and put in ears as ear drops.
* Pound fresh leaves of mango, *jamun*, cotton fruit and wood apple. Warm and put 2 or 3 drops in the ears for relief.
* Heat some sesame oil along with some garlic paste; filter and use warm as ear drops.

- Crush a few basil leaves and extract the juice. Pour 2 to 3 drops in each ear. This works as an antiseptic and anti-infective; it also provides relief.
- Heat the leaves of *sudarshan*, then crush to extract liquid. Put approx. 3 drops in each ear.
- Pound the roots of *bilva* and boil in mustard oil; filter, then use as ear drops.

NOSE BLEED

Ayurvedic Name *Nasagata Raktapitta, Nakseera*

Characteristic Symptoms
- Bleeding through the nose.
- If the blood is swallowed, coffee-ground vomitus is produced.
- Perhaps there may be signs of shock in case of prolonged or profuse bleeding.

Ayurvedic View
This ailment is caused by an aggravation or vitiation of the *pitta* or fire humor of the body.

Management by Home Cures
- Add *phitkari* to cow's milk and use as nasal drops.
- Apply a paste of *amla* into the scalp for relief.
- Pound 8 to 10 leaves of *sheesham*, add 1 tsp *mishri* and take with water 2 or 3 times a day.
- Hold a piece of ice on the head or bridge of the nose for some time.
- Chewing white onions and inhaling the fumes produced by burning them stops nasal bleeding.
- Pound a few flowers of pomegranate to extract the juice. Put approx. 2 drops of the juice in each nostril twice or thrice a day.
- Pound conch grass to extract fresh juice. Put in each nostril.

- Mix ½ tsp *phitkari* powder in a glass of cold buttermilk. Take this twice a day.
- A cloth dipped in *phitkari* water can be kept on the bridge of the nose for some time to control the bleeding.
- Crush fresh coriander to extract the juice. Use as nasal drops to control the bleeding.

FEVER
Ayurvedic Name   *Jwara*

Characteristic Symptoms
- Rise in the body temperature from the normal of 98.4 ° Fahrenheit or 37° Celsius.
- Perhaps rapid breathing and increase in the heart rate.
- Headache, backache, shivering, increased thirst and general lethargy.
- Febrile fits at high body temperature seen more commonly in children.

Ayurvedic View
According to Ayurveda, fever is caused by any of the 3 body humors, air, fire and phlegm. Other factors are vitiation of the vital fluid blood and climatic changes. This includes not only a rise in the body temperature, but also afflictions of the mind as well.

Management by Home Cures
- Pound 2 to 3 leaves of *tulsi* and add a few drops of ginger juice. Take 2 or 3 times a day with warm water or mixed in honey.
- Take 1 to 3 g powdered *ajwain* with warm water twice. This is useful in case of shivering along with fever.
- Take ¼ tsp pepper powder mixed with sugar and water 3 to 4 times a day.
- Make a decoction with *tulsi* leaves, black pepper, cloves and cinnamon. Take it warm 2 or 3 times with *mishri*.

- For fevers of mixed origin, take 1 to 3 g of the powder of large cardamom along with warm water twice a day.
- Prepare a decoction by boiling the stem of *giloy*. Allow to cool down gradually. Drink this potion 2 or 3 times with some sugar.
- Take 8 to 10 leaves of *tulsi* and 5 cloves. Boil these in 200 ml water till reduced to one-fourth; remove from flame and add *saindhav* salt. Take this drink 2 times.
- Pound dry coriander and mix into honey. Take in a dose of 3 to 5 g.
- Take a glass of hot milk mixed with ½ to 1 tsp turmeric powder.

GAS TROUBLE
Ayurvedic Name *Adhmana*

Characteristic Symptoms
- Belching, bloating or flatus.
- Pain in the abdomen in some cases.
- Expulsion of the wind may have offensive odour.

Ayurvedic View
An aggravation or vitiation of the *vatta* dosha or the air body humor is believed to be the prime cause of this ailment.

Management by Home Cures
- Pound dried ginger, *ajwain* and black salt and make a mixture taking equal parts of each. Take 1 g twice with warm water after meals.
- Take 2-3 cloves of garlic with warm water first thing in the morning.
- Sprinkle a few drops of fresh lemon juice on a piece of ginger and add black salt. Take it with meals for a few days.
- External application of *hing* on the umbilicus in case of abdominal discomfort caused by flatulence is recommended for infants and small children.
- When there is excessive production and expulsion of wind along with a foul smell, try this easy home remedy: Take 4 or 5 freshly ground peppercorns along with a

glassful of water mixed with a few drops of lemon, in the early morning on an empty stomach.
- Grate radish along with its leaves and extract the juice. Take approx. 30 ml once or twice.
- Pound a piece of cinnamom and boil in a glass of water. Take this drink lukewarm at least half an hour before meals.
- Hot fomentation of the stomach is recommended.
- Pound 1 to 2 g *hing* and mix in warm water; take approx. 20 ml twice.

HEADACHE

Ayurvedic Name *Shireshoola*

Characteristic Symptoms

- Pain in the head region that may get aggravated by any little stimulus.
- Perhaps severe and throbbing pain in severe cases.
- Relapses after intervals, as in case of migraine headache.

Ayurvedic View

Shireshoola is caused by both physical as well as psychic factors. All types of headaches are due to the imbalance of a particular body humor.

a. Due to vitiation of the air body humor.
b. Due to vitiation of the fire body humor.
c. Due to vitiation of the phlegm body humor.
d. Due to vitiation of all the 3 body humors.
e. When the headache is only on one side of the head it is called *ardhava bhedaka*.
f. The headache that increases and decreases with the movement of the sun is called *suryavarata*.
g. When the headache starts from the back of the head and migrates to the front and sides of the head this is known as *shankhaka*.
h. When the headache is acute and is difficult to treat it is called *anantavata*.

Management by Home Cures

- A local rub of warmed clove oil is a good handy cure for headache.
- Mix the powder of large cardamom in oil or balm and use it for local massage at the site of pain. This relieves associated symptoms of nasal congestion.
- Apply a paste made of *amla* and milk for headaches associated with heat stroke.
- Pound fresh or dry coriander into a paste and apply on the forehead for recurrent headaches.
- Make a paste of garlic in milk and add a few grains of salt. Apply the paste on the forehead.
- Use nasal drops of ghee in each nostril once or twice daily for chronic headache.
- Pound a few leaves of lemon to extract the juice and add to boiling hot water. Use for deep inhalation.
- As a cure for a nervous headache or headache caused by heatstroke, try this external application: Prepare a mixture of *gulab arka* and white *chandan* powder and apply it on the forehead.
- Pound a few *tulsi* leaves to extract the juice and rub 2 or 3 times a day.
- Soak a cloth in vinegar and place on the forehead.
- Chew fresh leaves of *tulsi* or inhale fresh *tulsi* juice mixed in boiling water. Or put the juice in the nostrils as nasal drops. This is soothing for the brain and relieves anxiety.
- Roast some *ajwain* and make into a poultice. Use this to make a hot fomentation on the forehead to relieve sinusitis.

- Massage the forehead with the juice of wheat grass or pour 2-3 drops in each nostril as nasal drops, especially for sinusitis.
- Pound 1 or 2 almonds in mustard oil and use to massage the neck, forehead and sides of the head.

HEART DISEASE
Ayurvedic Name   *Hridya Roga*

Characteristic Symptoms
- Decreased or no supply of oxygen and nutrient-rich blood to the heart muscle by the coronary artery results in the production of diseases like angina, myocardial infarction and coronary artery disease.
- Perhaps congenital or acquired diseases of the endocardium, myocardium and pericardium.

Ayurvedic View
Vitiation in the air body humor causes a disruption in the *rasa dhatu* of the body, which further results in production of heart disease. Any vitiation in the 3 humors, air, fire and phlegm, or distortion of all the humors, is believed to be the cause of heart disease.

Management by Home Cures
- Swallow 2 to 4 cloves of garlic on an empty stomach in the morning.
- Take powdered cloves 2 times a day.
- Powder of *ajwain* and *hing* can be taken twice after meals with water.
- Pound some bark of *arjun* and take ½ to 1 tsp of the powder 2 times along with milk or water.
- Boil 1 tsp of the powder of *arjun* bark in a mixture of 1 cup milk and 1 cup water till it is reduced to half. Take this twice a day.

- Take powdered cinnamon two times. This acts as a heart tonic and also helps to lower elevated cholesterol levels.
- Take 1 cup juice of freshly ground gourd; add 7 to 8 leaves each of *tulsi* and mint. Take the mixture 2 times.
- Massage on the chest with oil of eucalyptus is recommended.
- A regular intake of 3 to 5 g powdered asparagus or 10 to 20 ml asparagus juice is recommended for heart patients. It improves the overall functioning of this vital organ.
- Pound equal quantities of dried *amla* and *mishri* together. Take 1 to 2 tsp of the mixture twice a day along with water.
- Grapes are recommended because, being soft, slimy and cold by nature, grapes have a soothing and calming effect on the heart muscles.
- Prepare a decoction by boiling approx. 1 to 2 tsp dried ginger. Take it warm, once or twice a day.
- Take approx. 1 to 2 tsp fresh betel juice extracted by pounding betel leaves.
- A *murabba* (sweet jelly) of apple and carrot is recommended as a heart tonic.
- A moderate intake of ripe mangoes strengthens the heart and gives relief from palpitations.
- Take 3 to 6 g of the powdered seeds of lotus twice, to soothe and calm the heart.

HIGH BLOOD PRESSURE
Ayurvedic Name *Rakta Vaata, Uchch Raktachaap*

Characteristic Symptoms
- Rise in the systolic and/or diastolic blood pressures.
- Maybe headache, loss of sleep, palpitations, flushed face, easy fatigue and impaired digestion.
- There may be signs of increased urination.

Ayurvedic View
Vitiation of the *vatta* or the air body humor is believed to be the cause of this disease.

Management by Home Cures
- Asparagus taken in the form of powder or juice is used to combat high blood pressure.
- Swallow 2 to 3 fresh cloves of garlic daily on an empty stomach.
- A few drops of almond oil mixed in milk soothe the nerves and help to keep down the blood pressure caused by anxiety.
- Take approx. ½ tsp of the powder of the roots of *sarpgandha* twice or thrice.
- Take 1 to 3 g garlic paste along with buttermilk, twice.
- Take approx. 50 ml fresh juice of oranges twice daily.
- Roast garlic in a little *desi* ghee, then pound it. Take 1 to 3 g, 2 or 3 times a day.
- Boil the bark of the arjun tree to prepare a decoction. Take 30 ml twice a day.
- A *murrabba* (sweet jelly) of *aamla*, apple and carrots is recommended for controlling hypertension.

UTERINE PROLAPSE
Ayurvedic Name   *Yoni Vyapagata*

Characteristic Symptoms
- The uterus slips downwards in between the bowel and the bladder.
- It could be visible as it protrudes out of the vagina in advanced cases.

Ayurvedic View
It is believed that this disease is caused by vitiation in either or all of the 3 humors of the body, viz. air, fire and phlegm.

Management by Home Cures
- Boil mint leaves to prepare a decoction. Take approx. 50 ml twice daily.
- *Phitkari* mixed in water can be used as a douche.
- Pound the fresh leaves of *changaree* to extract the juice and take it twice. Or take ½ tsp of the dry powder of *changaree* leaves two times.
- Take approx. 3 to 5 g of the powder of *vacha* twice along with water or milk.
- Take ½ to 1 g powder of catechu twice.
- Boil catechu till reduced to one-fourth. Use this decoction as a douche.
- Pound approx. 10 to 15 leaves of *bala*, add some water and *mishri* and make into a drink. Take this potion twice.

- Knead 10 to 15 leaves of *bala* into the flour of *jaun*. Make chapattis out of this dough and take regularly for some days.
- A Sitz bath taken alternately with hot and cold water helps.

MOUTH ULCERS
Ayurvedic Name   *Mukh Paka*

Characteristic Symptoms
- Flat and shallow ulcers in the mouth with slightly raised margins.
- Acute pain and fever in severe cases.

Ayurvedic View
This disease is caused by vitation of the air, fire or phlegm humors of the body, leading to diffused inflammation and ulceration in the oral cavity. Vitiation of the *rakta* or blood is another cause. The aggravated fire or *pitta* humor of the body is a predisposing factor.

Management by Home Cures
- Local massage with powdered camphor 2 or 3 times daily helps. You could apply it plain or mixed with some glycerine.
- Prepare a mixture by pounding together rose petals, small cardamoms, cloves and *sheetal chini*. Mix into rose water and make into small balls. Keep 2 or 3 balls in the mouth 2 or 3 times a day.
- Mix 1 tsp ghee in ½ cup lukewarm milk. Use this mixture for gargles, then swallow it.
- Make a paste of garlic in coconut milk and apply it on the ulcers.
- Apply the milk of raw papaya on the ulcers.
- Apply the powder of catechu on the ulcers.

- Boil 2 tsp fennel in a glassful of water; add a piece of roasted *phitkari*. Use this as a mouth wash and for gargles.
- Use a decoction of liquorice both for gargles and swallowing.
- Make a paste of the leaves of *makoy* along with some buttermilk. Use this both for gargles and local application.
- Gargle with coconut milk, cold milk or buttermilk.
- *Phitkari* added to warm saline water can be used as a gargle and mouthwash.
- Take some powdered *phitkari* and mix it into glycerine; apply the paste on the ulcers.
- Take equal quantities of cumin seeds, large cardamom and *mishri* and pound them together. Take 3 to 5 g of this powder twice a day along with water.
- Use rose water mixed with glycerine as a local application on the ulcers.
- Boil some rose petals in a glassful of water till reduced to half. Gargle with this water every 4 hours.

WORM INFESTATION
Ayurvedic Name   *Udar Krimi*

Characteristic Symptoms
- Noted changes in the pattern of appetite (increase or decrease).
- Perhaps lethargy, drowsiness and listlessness.
- Occasional gastric upsets, prolonged irritant cough, occasional pain in the abdomen, loss of weight, shortness of breath, irritability, malnutrition and anaemia.

Ayurvedic View
Eating sweet and sour foods, eating during indigestion, and eating those foods that counteract each other results in the formation of worms. An aggravation of the *kapha dosha* is the predominant cause. These worms are:

a. Those that result from excessive production of phlegm in the stomach
b. Those that lie in the blood arteries or minute pores of the body and generally cause skin problems
c. Those which are formed in the bowels and lie in the large intestine

Management by Home Cures
- Take a mixture of some black pepper powder and black salt along with buttermilk 2 to 3 times for a few days.
- Take 10 to 20 ml *karela* juice mixed with some warm water.

- Pound mustard seeds into a powder. Take 1 to 4 g with warm water. Continue this therapy for a few days to get rid of the worms.
- Take the juice extracted from the bark of a *neem* tree with some honey.
- Take 1 to 2 tsp onion juice twice daily.
- Pound a few juvenile leaves of *neem* and make into a paste. Two to five g can be taken twice with warm water for a few days.
- Extract the milk from raw papaya and take 5 to 10 g of the milk with an equal amount of sugar or honey. This helps to combat roundworms.
- Boil the root bark of pomegranate to prepare a decoction. Boil 10 to 20 g of the decoction in a glassful of water and take preferably on an empty stomach to combat tapeworms. A mild laxative is generally recommended along with this remedy.
- Make a mixture with 1 tsp of the juice extracted by pounding *neem* leaves and 1 to 2 tsp of pure castor oil. Take at bedtime once or twice a month.
- Roast together some *ajwain* and jaggery. De-worm your children with 1 tsp of this sweet candy taken twice for a few days.
- Crush basil leaves to extract the juice. Mix approx. ½ tsp of the juice and approx. ½ to 1 tsp fresh lemon juice and take preferably on an empty stomach.
- Chewing *tulsi* leaves on an empty stomach daily for a few days fights recurrence of the worms.

- Take 1 to 3 g turmeric powder with warm water. For children ½ g is sufficient and this can be given mixed into some jaggery.

LOW BLOOD PRESSURE
Ayurvedic Name *Nyuna Raktachaap*

Characteristic Symptoms
- Decrease in the optimum blood pressure.
- Perhaps rapid pulse rate and cold sweats.
- Continuous feeling of weakness and sometimes giddiness.

Ayurvedic View
According to Ayurveda, low blood pressure results from vitiation of the vatta dosha or the air body humor.

Management by Home Cures
- Regular use of honey in the daily diet or honey mixed in milk helps to provide natural energy and works as a tonic for weakness.
- Pound approx. 1 tsp *shatavari* and *ashwagandha*, add ½ cup each milk and water and prepare a decoction. When the water evaporates, let the mixture cool gradually. Take this twice a day with sugar or honey.
- The ripe fruit of *bilva* is quite nutritious and a booster of vigour and energy. This can be crushed and made into a tasty drink by adding some sugar to it.
- Cardamom is a natural energy booster. Take 1 g cardamom powder with lukewarm milk.
- Grapes are invigorating and rejuvenating. Take fresh grapes or the juice extracted from them to boost up your energy levels.

- Groundnuts have most of the required nutrients and an unmatched source of protein. Roasted groundnuts are more nourishing. Soak the nuts overnight in some water for additional benefits. The sprouted nuts are a remarkable nutrition and energy supplement. Taking sprouted nuts regularly for some days may boost your blood pressure.
- Papaya is a natural source of a number of vitamins, minerals and digestive enzymes. You need to make it a regular supplement to your daily diet and feel the energy boost.
- Soak 10 to 15 dried grapes in water overnight. In the morning crush them along with the water and drink the potion. Repeat for a few days and feel the difference.
- Boil dates in sweetened milk. Take this milk warm along with the boiled dates, 2 or 3 times.
- Wheat grass is believed to be a wonderful elixir that rejuvenates and revitalizes the dormant energy levels. Extract the juice and consume it immediately while still fresh for best results.
- Sugarcane juice is also a good energy booster and recommended for low blood pressure.
- Take 2 to 4 g of *guggul* twice a day along with hot milk, preferably in the winter months.
- Take 100 g pulp of aloe vera and 1 kg milk; heat the mixture on a low flame till it thickens; add sugar to taste. Take 1 to 2 tsp twice. Continue for a few days to combat your low blood pressure.

HERNIA
Ayurvedic Name *Vrridhi Roga*

Characteristic Symptoms
- Pain in the mid-thoracic or epigastric region.
- Generally results from weakness in the abdominal wall.
- Perhaps enlargement of herniated sac during coughing, sneezing, etc.
- Occasional dysphagia and hiccough.
- Perhaps strangulation of the herniated sac.

Ayurvedic View
Vitiation in the body humors, air, fire and phlegm, or an imbalance in all the 3 humors causes this disease.

Management by Home Cures
- Take 4 leaves each of mango, *jamun*, *safeda* and *amrood*. Make a decoction in a glassful of water till reduced to one-fourth; remove from the flame, strain the mixture in a muslin cloth. This potion is to be taken twice.
- In the acute stage, it is advisable to fast on lemon water for a few days.

STOMACH ULCER
Ayurvedic Name *Grahani, Parinaam shool*

Characteristic Symptoms
- Burning sensation and distress in the epigastric region.
- Pain generally occurs just after taking food.
- Tenderness in the epigastric region.

Ayurvedic View
Stomach ulcer is believed to be a consequence of aggravation in the air body humor, beyond its normal limits. Vitiation in the fire humor is often the collateral cause.

Management by Home Cures
- Take 3 to 5 g powdered *mulathee* along with cow's milk.
- Take 100 to 500 ml coconut water twice or thrice a day.
- Take ½ cup juice of beetroot mixed with 1 tsp honey.
- Take 1 to 3 g powdered *aamla* 2 or 3 times along with water.
- Use the fresh pulp of the fruit of *bilva* in case of gastric or peptic ulcers.
- Soak 2 to 5 leaves of *bael* overnight. In the morning crush them and drink the water.
- Take approx. 30 ml cabbage juice twice or thrice daily.
- Pound 5 g mixture of liquorice, sesame seeds and dried ginger along with some jaggery. Mix in milk and take it 2 times.
- Make the seeds of *bilva* into a dry powder. Take 1 to 2 g two or three times along with buttermilk.

WOUND
Ayurvedic Name *Vrana*

Characteristic Symptoms
- Pain and bleeding due to a cut or opening in the skin.
- Perhaps presence of exposed tissues.

Ayurvedic View
Vrana is considered in Ayurveda as a conjuncture that tears off the body. As per the predominance of the *doshas*, the wounds have been categorized as *Vattaja, Pittaja, Kaphaja* and Raktaja Vrana.

Management by Home Cures
- Local application of *phitkari* powder at the site of the injury arrests blood loss and gives antiseptic cover as well.
- Sprinkle some powder of camphor on the site to combat inflammation, blood loss and pain and to prevent degeneration of the wound.
- Crush the fruit of *aamla* to extract the juice. Take approx. 50 ml two or three times a day.
- Smoke from the leaves of the margosa tree can be applied onto an open wound; this acts as a natural antiseptic and insecticide.
- When there is a possibility of an internal wound or injury, it is advisable as a first aid to take a glass of hot milk mixed with approx. ½ tsp powdered *phitkari* and ½ tsp turmeric powder. This could prevent the

complications arising from any hidden blood loss inside the body.
- An application of turmeric warmed with some mustard oil can treat pain and swelling resulting from a wound. Turmeric also has unique wound-healing properties. Besides, it prevents blood loss from the site. It is also advisable to drink hot milk with a teaspoon of turmeric added to it.

TOOTH ACHE AND BLEEDING GUMS
Ayurvedic Name *Danta Roga, Dantaveshta*

Characteristic Symptoms
- Pain in the teeth generally due to dental caries.
- The gums are swollen and spongy and bleed on touching.
- Perhaps foul odour.

Ayurvedic View
Tooth and gum disorders are a consequence of weak digestion and lack of oral hygiene.

Management by Home Cures
- Regular massage with powdered black pepper on the teeth and gums relieves pain and also prevents frequent dental problems.
- For toothache, degradation of the teeth or bleeding gums, try a massage with the powder of camphor.
- A local massage of the powder of catechu is an effective cure for spongy and bleeding gums, mouth ulcers and gingivitis.
- In case of dental caries and toothache, apply 1 or 2 drops of cinnamom oil to a piece of cotton and press into the cavity.
- Press a clove between the teeth or press cotton dipped in clove oil into the dental crevice. This relieves the pain and has germicidal properties as well.

- Use a mixture of ginger juice and honey as a local application.
- Prepare a decoction from the bark of the mango tree and use as a gargle to cure dental ailments like tooth decay, bleeding from the teeth and bad breath.
- Dry the seed of the mango and make into a paste. This paste, when massaged into the teeth and gums, stops the bleeding instantly.
- Powdered *phitkari* can be rubbed onto the gums and teeth to keep them clear of the problems of spongy and bleeding gums and toothache. You could also gargle with *phitkari* dissolved in water.

DECREASED LACTATION
Ayurvedic Name *Nyun Satanya*

Characteristic Symptoms
- Decreased or no production of milk.
- Insufficient milk production is not able to satisfy the need of the infant.

Ayurvedic View
Vitiation in the air, fire or phlegm humors of the body or an imbalance in all the 3 *doshas* is the cause of this ailment.

Management by Home Cures
- Asparagus stimulates an increase in milk production. Pound the roots of the asparagus to make a powder. Take 1 to 2 tsp, 2 or 3 times along with a glassful of milk.
- Take 30 ml of the juice extracted from the fresh roots of asparagus twice.
- Clove is also approved for lactating mothers because it sanitizes and increases milk production.
- Chew fennel, or take the powder, or boil it in sweetened milk.
- Groundnuts enhance the production and nutrition content of milk. Roasted groundnuts can be added to jaggery and cooked on a slow flame along with some ghee. Add roasted cumin seeds, fennel, thyme and dried ginger powder for increased benefits. Take this dessert twice after meals.

- *Methi* enhances the milk production and is a natural uterine contractor. It is advised after delivery.
- Boil the tubers of *vidari* to prepare a decoction. Take approx. 30 ml, twice a day.
- Lactating mothers need to supplement their daily diet with papaya and fresh juice of sugarcane.

SWELLING
Ayurvedic Name *Shoth*

Characteristic Symptoms
- Non-inflammatory swelling anywhere in the body.
- Accumulation of water inside the body tissues that may present as a pit or depression on pressing on a bony structure.
- May be localized or may affect whole limbs or large part of the body like the abdomen.

Ayurvedic View
Shoth roga emerges from vitiation in the air humor, which causes an imbalance in the fire, phlegm and the blood. This further causes accumulation of fluid in the skin tissues and produces swelling in the body.

Management by Home Cures
- Mix powdered dried ginger into some sesame oil and massage into the swelling.
- Apply a hot paste of onion on the site.
- Pound the fresh leaves of *bilva* to extract the juice. Take approx. 10 to 20 ml, two to three times to reduce pain and swelling.
- Mix some turmeric powder in the pulp of aloe vera, heat the mixture on low heat then tie it in a cloth; apply warm on the site of the swelling. Or apply the paste locally on the swollen area.

- Pound *punarnava* to extract the fresh juice. Take 20 ml two or three times a day.
- Add camphor to mustard oil, sesame seed oil or any medicated oil and use to reduce swelling and pain.
- A hot paste of *methi* when applied locally to an abscess or swelling on the body can provide immediate relief.
- Apply turmeric warmed along with some mustard oil to treat any pain and swelling resulting from an injury.

DEPRESSION
Ayurvedic Name *Avsaada*

Characteristic Symptoms
- Lack of interest in small pleasures; obvious mood changes.
- Feeling of misery, restlessness and loss of sleep.
- Impairment of digestion; constipation and loss of hunger.
- Perhaps suicidal attempts in case of severe depression.

Ayurvedic View
Vitiation in the humors of the body, *vatta*, *pitta* and *kapha*, and also imbalance in the mental states of *rajasa* and *tamasa* are the predominant causes of this disease.

Management by Home Cures
- Mix 1 tsp powdered asparagus into ½ tsp honey. Take it twice daily along with warmed cow's milk. It fights depression and works as a brain tonic.
- Extract the fresh juice of *bramhi* and take 10 to 20 ml twice a day.
- A regular intake of honey helps to fight stress and feelings of depression.
- Take *amla* in the form of fresh juice, powder, or jelly, as a tonic to remove mental and physical fatigue. It rejuvenates and revitalises the entire body system.
- Shallow-fry some *brahmi* leaves in *desi* ghee; add pepper and some sugar: Take this mixture regularly.

- Add honey and a few drops of almond oil to the powders of *brahmi* and *shankhpushpi*. Take approx. 3 to 5 g once or twice daily.
- Powder the root of liquorice and take it with honey and ghee (in unequal quantities). This works as a general as well as brain tonic and helps fight anxiety and depression.
- Pound approx. 1 large tsp dry coriander seeds. Remove the husk and boil the seeds in a glassful of milk. Add some sugar and take this, preferably at bedtime.
- Dry *bramhi* in the shade and make it into a powder. Take 1 tsp with milk once or twice a day.
- Saffron is believed to be a boon for the brain as well as the entire nervous system. Add a pinch of saffron to milk and take it at bedtime.
- *Petha* has a calming and cooling effect on the brain and the entire nervous system. Take approx. 20 to 30 ml *petha* juice twice a day on an empty stomach.

SORE THROAT

Characteristic Symptoms
- May be accompanied by fever with pain on swallowing.
- The pharynx gets red and inflamed.
- Enlarged and tender lymph nodes may be present.

Ayurvedic View
Vitiation of *vatta, pitta* or *kapha doshas* or imbalance of all the 3 humors causes this disease.

Management by Home Cures
- Massage the throat externally with camphor added to mustard oil. This relieves a sore throat.
- Catechu causes a decrease in phlegm or *kapha* body humor Take ½ to 1 g of catechu twice, mixed with honey.
- Chew slowly on some onion bulbs mixed with a little jaggery and slowly swallow the juice.
- Take saline water gargles or gargles of warm, salted black tea.
- Boil some *tulsi* leaves in water and make into a decoction. Drink this and gargle with it as well.
- Cinnamom is also a destroyer of phlegm and is recommended for a sore throat. Take 2 to 3 g cinnamom powder mixed with 1 tsp honey. For better relief add a pinch of black pepper powder and a few drops of ginger juice.

- Try gargles with the juice of wheat grass and drink it as well.
- Gargles with a decoction prepared by boiling the bark of the pomegranate tree is recommended 2 or 3 times a day.

WHOOPING COUGH

Ayurvedic Name *Dusht Kasa, Kukkar Kasa*

Characteristic Symptoms

- Sneezing, watering of eyes, throat irritation, mild cough and loss of hunger initially.
- Later, paroxysms of coughing that end in a high-pitched 'whoop' sound usually accompanied by vomiting.
- Severity of paroxysms and a series of rapid and violent expiratory coughs, which at times leave the patient blue in the face.

Ayurvedic View

This disease is caused by a distortion in the *vatta* or the air humor of the body.

Management by Home Cures

- Pound fresh ginger to extract the juice. Mix approx. 1 to 2 tsp in an equal amount of honey and take twice a day.
- Boil approx. ½ to 1 tsp powder of *pippali* in a cup of cow's milk mixed with a cup of water till reduced to one-fourth. Take it warm mixed with some *mishri* or honey.
- Burn *apamarg* and collect the ashes; mix the ashes in honey and take approx. 1 g, two or three times.
- Pound 2 to 4 leaves of betel and basil and a piece of ginger together and extract the juice. Take ½ to 1 tsp mixed with an equal amount of honey.
- Mix ¼ to ½ tsp roasted and pounded *phitkari* in an equal amount of powdered *mishri*. Take this mixture 2 or 3 times with some warm water.

CRAMPS
Ayurvedic Name *Khalani, Mamasagata Vayu*

Characteristic Symptoms
- Painful and spasmodic contractions of muscles.
- Generally muscles of the limbs, particularly the calf muscles are affected.
- Maybe an indication of any other disease in the body.

Ayurvedic View
This condition is caused by a deposit or blockage in the nerve and muscle tissues by metabolic wastes. Vitiation in the air body humor adds to the predisposing cause.

Management by Home Cures
- A massage with sesame oil or mustard oil on the affected area is recommended.
- Take a hot glassful of cow's milk mixed with ¼ tsp dried ginger powder and 1 tsp turmeric powder at bedtime.
- Take 1 to 2 tsp castor oil at bedtime.
- Extract juice of the fresh fruit of *amla*. Take 20 ml twice a day.
- Pound the roots of *ashwagandha* to make a powder. Take approx 5 g daily with milk. This works as a nerve tonic.
- Apply a hot fomentation on the affected area with a bag of salt or sand.
- Powder the seeds of *erand* and take with milk, or boil in milk and take 2 or 3 times.
- Boil 1 tsp sesame seeds in milk and take it warm at bedtime.
- Stretching exercises of the limbs are beneficial.

HICCOUGH
Ayurvedic Name *Hikka Roga*

Characteristic Symptoms
- Spasmodic drawing in of air into the lungs causing a click sound due to sudden closure of vocal cords.
- May result from digestive disorders.

Ayurvedic View
This disease is caused by an aggravation and upward movement of the *vatta* or the air body humor. Other causes include weak digestion, inappropriate diet as well as inappropriate method of eating. Some psychological factors like anger, nervousness and anxiety may be additional causes.

Management by Home Cures
- Sucking on a piece of ginger is recommended.
- With the onset of hiccoughs, try taking ½ to 1 tsp honey instantly.
- Gulp down mouthfuls of plain water during the onset of hiccoughs.
- Boil 4 or 5 cardamoms in a glass of water to make a decoction. Take 2 or 3 times.
- Ash produced by burning approx. 0.125 g peacock's feathers can be taken 2 or 3 times.
- Sometimes psychological intervention is required to direct the mind towards some other engrossing situation.

- Chew 2 or 3 cloves for some time followed by a glass of water.
- Take 1 or 2 pinches of the ash of cardamom 2 or 3 times, mixed into honey or with some warm water.
- Inhale the fumes of a burnt piece of *hing*.

CERVICAL SPONDYLITIS

Ayurvedic Name *Griva Sandhigata Vatta, Manyastambha*

Characteristic Symptoms
- Pain and stiffness in the region of the neck, shoulder and arm.
- There may be restrictive movements of the neck.
- Perhaps vertigo, which is often aggravated on touching the chin to the chest.

Ayurvedic View
Vitiation or aggravation in the *vatta* and *kapha* humors is the predisposing cause.

Management by Home Cures
- Mix 1 tsp of the powder of raw turmeric and ¼ tsp dried ginger powder into a glass of warm milk and take at bedtime.
- Massage the back of the neck with warmed sesame oil or mustard oil, or some medicated muscle relaxant oil or balm.
- Apply a hot fomentation on the neck with the help of a sand or salt poultice.
- Prepare a decoction of dried ginger and add some pure castor oil. Take approx. ½ cup, warmed, at bedtime.
- Dissolve some camphor in mustard oil and warm it. Apply tolerably hot and massage into the site of pain.
- Neck exercises and Accupressure are recommended.
- Mix dried ginger powder in warmed mustard oil and massage into the back of the neck. Take a hot fomentation afterwards.

COUGH
Ayurvedic Name *Kasa Roga*

Characteristic Symptoms
- Bouts of cough that may be short, half-suppressed or exhausting.
- The cough may be dry, wet or allergic.
- Perhaps acute or chronic.

Ayurvedic View
Vitiated *vatta* or air movement towards the upper part of the neck and head region producing the sound of torn bamboo. According to the vitiated humor, cough or Kasa is categorized as *vattaja, pittaja* and *kaphaja* type. Other than these, there are 2 more types: *kshataja kasa* is produced by injury, and *kshayaja kasa* which is a consequence of vitiation of all the 3 humors of the body.

Management by Home Cures
- Pound black pepper and jaggery together and make into small balls. Hold 1 or 2 of these in the mouth during bouts of coughing and slowly suck on them.
- Make a decoction by boiling *tulsi* leaves with moderate quantities of ginger and black pepper. Take it warm, mixed with 1 tsp honey, twice or thrice a day.
- Chew 2 or 3 leaves of holy basil, two or three times.
- Take 2 to 3 black peppercorns; add a few cumin seeds and some salt. Pound the ingredients together and take twice along with warm water.

- Pound 1 or 2 cardamoms to make a powder and mix with honey; for better results add equal quantities of freshly ground pepper and dried ginger powder. Take approx. ¼ to ½ tsp, 2 to 3 times.
- Suck on a piece of the dried roots of liquorice. Or take approx. ½ tsp powdered liquorice with a spoonful of honey twice.
- In case of a dry cough, to lubricate your throat, take a glassful of warm milk mixed with ½ to 1 tsp (5-10 drops) almond oil or ½ tsp ghee.

IMPOTENCE
Ayurvedic Name *Klaivya*

Characteristic Symptoms
- Inability to perform the sexual act.
- Perhaps incomplete performance.

Ayurvedic View
This disease is believed to arise from vitiation of any of the 3 *doshas* of the body, *vatta, pitta* and *kapha*, or by distortion of all the 3 humors.

Management by Home Cures
- 5 to 10 ml fresh juice of ginger or 1 to 2 g dried ginger powder has an aphrodisiac effect.
- 1 to 3 g of powdered onion seeds can be taken twice daily.
- Regular intake of *guggul* and its medicinal formulations are quite beneficial.
- Take the powdered seeds of *kaunch* along with honey and milk twice a day.
- Take hot *urad* dal regularly, with a spoonful of *desi* ghee added to it.
- Pound the dried roots of *ashwagandha* to make a powder. Take 3 to 6 g along with milk once or twice daily.
- Coconut can be taken in unlimited quantities.
- Fresh sugarcane or pomegranate juice is recommended.
- Pound the dried rhizome of *safed musli*: Take 3 to 6 g twice along with milk.
- Take 1 to 2 g powdered basil seeds along with milk, twice.
- *Shilajit* is another efficient drug of choice.

HYSTERIA

Ayurvedic Name *Yoshapsmara*

Characteristic Symptoms
- The symptoms are generally self-oriented.
- Convulsive fits, contractions of the limbs, temporary loss of sensation over areas of the body.
- Somatic and psychological symptoms but without lesions.
- Multiple personality behaviour.

Ayurvedic View
This disease is considered a form of epilepsy.

Management by Home Cures
- Massage sesame oil into the scalp and on the soles of the feet.
- Soak approx. 5 almonds in water overnight. In the morning remove the skins and crush into a paste. Mix the paste with an equal amount of pounded *mishri* and take daily on an empty stomach.
- Take approx. 1 tsp powdered *vacha* with milk twice daily.
- Pound garlic to make a paste. Sniff this during an attack of hysteria for relief from the symptoms.
- Take approx. 1 tsp powdered *shatavari* along with approx. 20 ml of the juice of *bramhi* twice. Either of the herbs taken alone has a good effect on the intellect.
- Pound a few cloves of garlic and extract the juice. Filter through a muslin cloth and use as ear drops.

- This being more of a perceptual ailment, the patient should seek psychological counselling and adopt a positive attitude along with trying the above cures.

HEAT STROKE
Ayurvedic Name *Daah Roga*

Characteristic Symptoms
- Redness, swelling or blister formation on the parts of the body exposed to rays of the sun or excessive heat.
- Burning sensation, itching, pain and tenderness.
- Contact with clothing may be uncomfortable.

Ayurvedic View
An aggravation or vitiation in the fire or the *pitta dosha* causes this disease.

Management by Home Cures
- Apply a paste of sandalwood over the affected areas.
- Apply a paste prepared by pounding *isabgol* in water.
- Local application of the juice of onion is recommended.
- Apply curd (yogurt) over the affected parts of the body. Leave to dry, then wash with cold water. Repeat this as often as required.
- Sandalwood syrup, rose syrup or cooled and sweetened fresh lime can be taken 2 or 3 times a day for internal cooling.

DYSENTERY
Ayurvedic Name *Raktatisar*

Characteristic Symptoms
- Blood and mucous in small frequent loose stools.
- May be accompanied by abdominal pain; tenesmus, sometimes fever and dehydration in advanced cases.
- General malaise, coated tongue, listlessness and restlessness.

Ayurvedic View
This disease is believed to result from an aggravation of the *pitta* or fire humor of the body. Vitiation in the *pitta dosha* distorts the blood or *rakta dhatu* and causes the disease.

Management by Home Cures
- Extract the pulp from the raw fruit of *bilva* and roast it on a fire. Mix into an equal quantity of jaggery or honey and take 2 or 3 times.
- Take approx. 1 tsp of the dried powder of *bilgiri* with honey twice a day.
- An infusion prepared from lemon and taken on an empty stomach is recommended.
- Mix *isabgol* powder with curd (yogurt) and some roasted, crushed cumin seeds. Take 2 or 3 times a day.
- The seeds of *isabgol*, when roasted, tend to bind the loose stools and are recommended.
- A powder prepared from the dried flowers of the mango tree is recommended.

TYPHOID
Ayurvedic Name *Aantrik jwara*

Characteristic Symptoms
- Presence of low grade fever lasting for more than 5 days.
- Perhaps diarrhoea accompanied by headache and general malaise.
- In more advanced cases, fever may rise to alarming heights along with signs of dehydration.
- Perhaps loss of appetite and brown and furred tongue.

Ayurvedic View
According to Ayurveda, typhoid fever is a combined result of vitiation of all the 3 body humors.

Management by Home Cures
- Take coconut water 3 or 4 times a day.
- Pound a few fresh leaves of mint as well as Holy basil. Take approx 1 tsp of each and mix together. Take this thrice a day with some *mishri* powder or honey.
- Take approx. 20 ml of a decoction prepared by boiling a few leaves of Holy basil 2 or 3 times.
- Boil a stick of cinnamom along with a few black peppercorns to prepare a decoction. Take approx. 20 ml, warmed, preferably with a teaspoon of honey or *mishri* powder.

PNEUMONIA

Ayurvedic Name *Shwasanak Jwara*

Characteristic Symptoms
- Fever with shivering, painful cough, stabbing pain in the chest and perhaps respiratory distress.
- Rust-coloured or blood-stained sputum.

Ayurvedic View
Pneumonia is believed to result from vitiation of the *vatta* or air body humor.

Management by Home Cures
- Take 5 to 10 ml of the fresh juice of ginger, or take 1 to 2 g dried ginger powder, 2 times daily.
- Take honey mixed in a glass of lukewarm water 2 or 3 times a day.
- Pound 2 to 4 bulbs of garlic and mix into the same amount of honey. Take this mixture twice daily for a rapid cure.
- Pound a few mint leaves and extract the juice. Take 1 tsp 3 or 4 times with a teaspoon of honey.
- Massage the chest with warmed turpentine oil mixed with some camphor.

LEPROSY
Ayurvedic Name *Kushta Roga*

Characteristic Symptoms
- Pale-coloured, non-itchy patch on the skin along with loss of sensation.
- Perhaps erosion of tissues due to repeated injuries in the areas of decreased sensation.
- Perhaps non-sensitive macules or nodules leading to formation of ulcers and necrosis.
- Later on extensive disfigurement and deformity.

Ayurvedic View
This disease is believed to result from distortion of all the 3 body humors. Leprosy has been further categorized into seven types of *maha kushta* and eleven types of *kshudra kushta*.

Management by Home Cures
- Apply a paste of catechu prepared by pounding it in water.
- Extract the juice from wheat grass. Take approx. 50 ml twice a day and also apply it on the affected skin.
- Wash the area with a decoction prepared by boiling a few leaves of *neem*.
- Take 2 or 3 juvenile leaves of *neem*. Pound them along with 2 or 3 black peppercorns and make into small balls. Take one or two balls on an empty stomach twice.

* Local application of turmeric paste as well as taking 1 tsp turmeric powder mixed in milk twice a day is recommended.
* Wash the area with a decoction of *neem* and the 3 *myrobalans*.

STERILITY
Ayurvedic Name *Vandhyatva*

Characteristic Symptoms
- Inability to conceive among females.
- Perhaps presence of congenital defects.
- Maybe functional in some cases.

Ayurvedic View
Vitiation in any of the 3 body humors or a combined distortion of all the 3 *doshas* is the cause of this disease.

Management by Home Cures
- Take approx. 3 to 5 g powdered seeds of holy basil twice a day preferably on an empty stomach.
- Swallow 2 to 4 cloves of garlic in the morning on an empty stomach along with cow's milk.
- Crush the roots of asparagus to extract the fresh juice. Take approx. 20 ml twice.
- Take approx. 50 ml of the fresh juice extracted by pounding wheat grass 3 times a day.
- Powder the roots of *ashwagandha*. Take 3 to 5 g twice.
- Dry the roots of the banyan tree in the shade and pound into powder. Take approx. 3 g of the powder along with milk after the cessation of the menstrual cycle for a period of 3 days.
- Pound the roots of asparagus to make a powder. Take 3 to 5 g twice a day with milk.
- Take approx. 3 g powdered seeds of *shivlingi* on an empty stomach twice a day.

THINNESS
Ayurvedic Name *Kryshata*

Characteristic Symptoms
- Debilitated and undernourished appearance along with general weakness.
- Skin of the body, particularly the hips, stomach and neck region, has little or no fat deposits.
- Bones and joints visible and the veins visibly protruding all over the body.

Ayurvedic View
This disease is a consequence of a number of factors: A diet of dry food, lack of nutrition and over exerting the body and the mind. Heredity, old age and prolonged illness also add to this condition.

Management by Home Cures
- Regular massage of the body with coconut oil in summer, and mustard or sesame oil in winter is advised.
- Prepare a *halwa* (dessert) of almonds. Take warm 3 or 4 times daily.
- Increase the intake of milk and milk products, ghee and sweet foods.
- Pound the dried roots of *ashwagandha*. Take 1 to 2 tsp of this powder twice daily along with a glass of sweetened milk.
- Take 3 to 5 g powdered asparagus mixed in a teaspoon of ghee twice a day followed by a glassful of sweetened warm milk.

- Ground *musali* can be boiled in milk and taken twice.
- Mix together the fresh juice extracted from carrots, spinach leaves and turnips and take approx. 100 ml twice.
- The patient is advised to develop a carefree attitude and sleep soundly.

ITCHING
Ayurvedic Name *Kandu*

Characteristic Symptoms
* Itching, scratching and rubbing on the skin.
* Feeling of malaise, anxiety and sleeplessness in advanced cases.

Ayurvedic View
The cause of this malady is aggravation or vitiation of the phlegm humor of the body.

Management by Home Cures
* Prepare a powder out of equal parts of fennel and dry coriander. Add double the quantity of powdered *mishri*. Take approx. 3 to 5 g of this powder twice daily for some days.
* Make a paste with the powder of catechu and water and apply to the site of itching.
* Apply some sandalwood oil mixed into some coconut oil or sesame oil and massage into the affected areas.
* Apply the juice of lemon and juice of basil mixed together.
* Apply wheat grass juice onto the affected skin and also take 50 ml twice daily. It acts as a blood purifier and natural antiseptic.
* Pound some raw turmeric and make into powder. Take ½ to 1 tsp twice, preferably mixed in a glass of milk.
* Apply turmeric mixed in mustard oil or coconut oil at the site of itching.

SCABIES
Ayurvedic Name *Kachchhu*

Characteristic Symptoms
- Itchy vesicular eruptions on the skin.
- The itching is worse at night.
- Perhaps inflammation, scratching and pus formation.
- Presence of characteristic burrows.

Ayurvedic View
This disease is believed to result from vitiation in all the 3 body humors, *vatta, pitta* and *kapha* with aggravation of the phlegm humor of the body.

Management by Home Cures
- Boil the bark of the *neem* tree to prepare a decoction. Apply locally on the affected skin.
- Prepare a paste of *neem* leaves and mix with some turmeric powder and mustard oil. Apply this on the affected areas and leave on for at least one hour.
- Apply camphor mixed in coconut oil at the site of the lesions.
- Mix sulphur into ghee and heat on low flame till all the sulphur is almost burnt; remove from the heat and allow it to cool gradually. Apply locally once or twice a day.
- Extract the juice by crushing a few mint leaves; apply locally.

MEASLES
Ayurvedic Name *Romantika*

Characteristic Symptoms
- Fever, headache, general malaise, cough and cold, conjunctivitis, photophobia and discharge from the eyes are early symptoms.
- Koplick spots emerge on the mucous membranes.
- Perhaps on the 4th day of the fever, a characteristic rash appears, starting from the face and behind the ears, and later spreads all over the body.

Ayurvedic View
This disease is believed to result from vitiation in both the fire and phlegm humors of the body.

Management by Home Cures
- Pound some leaves of tamarind and take twice a day.
- Soak 1 tsp each of coriander and cumin seeds in ½ glass water overnight. In the morning mash them, add *mishri* and drink the water.
- Mix some cow's ghee in cow's milk. Add *mishri* and take it twice daily for some days.
- Pound a piece of liquorice to make a powder. Take approx. ¼ to ½ tsp either with water or mixed in 1 tsp honey.
- Pound together a few tamarind leaves and a piece of raw turmeric. Mix this paste in water and take the drink 2 or 3 times.

- Prepare a mixture with the powders of cloves and liquorice. Take this in a dose of 3 to 6 g twice, preferably mixed with a teaspoon of honey or with warm water.
- Soak some raisins in water overnight. Take these in the morning on an empty stomach.

MENTAL AILMENT
Ayurvedic Name *Mastishka Vikara*

Characteristic Symptoms
- False beliefs, suspicion, oppression and hallucinations.
- Attempts at suicide and homicide, disregard of personal appearance, tearing of clothes or extravagant dressing.
- Obsessive stealing, refusal of food and drinks, indecent exposure of self.

Ayurvedic View
Vitiation in any of the 3 *doshas* or body humors, *vatta* (air), *pitta* (fire) and *kapha* (phlegm) causes this disease.
1. Vitiation in the air humor destroys mental balance and gives rise to grief and infatuation.
2. When the fire increases inside the body, it produces states of excessive fear, lust and grief.
3. Similarly, imbalance in the phlegm humor causes lethargy and anxiety.
4. Another cause is an imbalance in *rajas* and *tamas*. These 2 states are ascribed to *iccha* (desire) and *dwesh* (repulsion). When they cross the limits set by social norms and values or excite the *doshas* or basic humors of the body, the result is a degeneration of brain power and the birth of mental diseases.

Management by Home Cures
- Soak a few almonds in water overnight. In the morning remove the skins and pound into a paste. Mix the

almond paste in a glass of milk and boil for some time; allow it to cool gradually. Take this drink with some *mishri* added to it twice daily.
- *Amla* can be taken in the form of fresh juice, in powdered form or even as a sweet *amla* jelly.
- Mix 1 tsp powdered asparagus into ½ tsp honey. Take twice daily along with warmed cow's milk to fight mental stress and weakness.
- Shallow-fry some *brahmi* leaves in *desi* ghee. Add freshly ground pepper and some *mishri*. Take this mixture regularly as it promotes the powers of the brain.
- Extract the juice from fresh *bramhi* and take 10 to 20 ml once or twice daily.
- Take 1 tsp powdered vacha with cow's milk twice a day.
- To the powder of *brahmi* and *shankhpushpi* add honey and a few drops of almond oil. Regular intake will boost your mental powers and help fight stress.
- Powdered root of liquorice when taken with honey and ghee (both in unequal quantities) works as a brain tonic and helps fight everyday stress.
- *Petha* has a calming and cooling effect on the brain and the entire nervous system, and strengthens brain power.

FILARIASIS

Ayurvedic Name *Shilipada Jwara*

Characteristic Symptoms

- Recurrent episodes of fever along with inflammation of lymph glands.
- Perhaps urticaria, inflammation of the testicles, arthritis and gross enlargement of the legs.
- The inflammation tends to increase, and in advanced cases the legs resemble those of an elephant and there is difficulty in walking.

Ayurvedic View

This disease is a result of the vitiation of all the 3 body humors, particularly the kapha or phlegm.

Management by Home Cures

- Take approx. ½ tsp dried ginger powder with warm water twice a day.
- Mix some turmeric powder and jaggery in warm water or purified cow's urine. Take 2 to 3 times per day.

DIPTHERIA
Ayurvedic Name *Rohini*

Characteristic Symptoms
- Sore throat, fever and exudation of the membrane on the tonsils and back of pharynx.
- Formation of greyish-white membrane on tonsils and wall of the pharynx which, on removing forcibly, re-emerges and leaves behind bleeding surfaces.
- Perhaps high pitched cough, loss of breath and a feeling of choking and suffocation.

Ayurvedic View
The cause of this disease is the vitiation in the *vatta*, *pitta* or *kapha doshas* or an imbalance of all the 3 humors.

Management by Home Cures
- Extract the juice from basil by pounding a few leaves; add ginger juice and freshly ground black pepper. Take 1 to 2 tsp of this mixture 2 or 3 times with an equal quantity of honey added to it.
- Take 3 to 6 g of the powdered dried roots of liquorice along with warm water or mixed in honey.
- Prepare a decoction with the seeds of *methi* and use it warm for gargles 2 or 3 times.
- Extract the juice of betel by pounding the leaves. Take this twice or thrice a day mixed in honey.

- Pound 2 or 3 bulbs of garlic and a little jaggery together. Heat the mixture on a low flame and take it warm twice daily.
- The milk from a raw papaya may be used as throat paint.
- Gargle every 4 to 6 hours with *phitkari* mixed in water.
- Boil 2 to 5 bulbs of garlic in a cup each of milk and water till one-fourth remains. Remove from flame and allow to cool gradually. Take it warm once or twice a day (preferably at bedtime) with a teaspoon of *mishri* or honey added to it.
- Take approx. 3 g powdered raw turmeric twice along with warm water.
- Massage the chest and throat with warmed mustard oil mixed with 1 tsp roasted *ajwain*.

FUNGAL INFECTION
Ayurvedic Name *Dadru*

Characteristic Symptoms
- Circular lesions, which are itchy, scaly and clear in the centre and may occur on any exposed area of the body.
- Perhaps itchy lesions in the axillae and under the breast in females.
- Perhaps baldness, itching and scaling in the scalp; the hair becomes dry and brittle.
- Ringworm sometimes infects the inner and upper parts of the thighs and the groins.
- There may be dryness, rigidity and discolouration of the nails and formation of black streaks on the nail surfaces.

Ayurvedic View
Vitiation in the 3 *doshas* of the body, particularly aggravation of the *pitta* and *kapha doshas* causes this skin disease which is categorized as a variety of *kshudra kushta*.

Management by Home Cures
- For skin disorders of fungal origin, rub the juice of garlic on the site of the infection.
- Pound a piece of fresh, raw turmeric along with a few basil leaves. Use this paste as a local application twice a day.
- Pound together a few *neem* leaves and raw turmeric to make a paste. Apply this at the site of infection 2 or 3 times.

- Pound the seeds of *chakkermard* to make a paste and mix it into the juice of radish. Apply this paste on the affected areas.
- In case of skin rash with fungal infection, make a paste out of freshly ground basil leaves and apply locally.
- Local application of mint juice is also recommended.
- Mix camphor in some coconut oil. Apply on the skin patch daily at least 3 times.

ULCERATIVE COLITIS
Ayurvedic Name   *Adhog Rakta Pitta*

Characteristic Symptoms
- Loose motions with blood.
- Low grade fever, pain in lower abdomen usually on left side, loss of hunger and loss of weight in long-lasting cases.
- Perhaps tenderness along the course of the colon.
- Frequent recurrences and remissions.

Ayurvedic View
This disease is the result of vitiation in the fire or *pitta dosha* which further causes a distortion in the blood or the *rakta dhatu*. When this impure blood escapes from the body through the lower orifice, it is said to be adhog *rakta pitta*.

Management by Home Cures
- Take 1 to 2 tsp powdered dried seeds of *bilva* twice or thrice along with buttermilk.
- Extract the pulp from the fresh fruit of *bilva* and take 2 or 3 times.
- The infusion prepared from lemon and taken on an empty stomach is another useful remedy.
- Take *isabgol* mixed with curd (yogurt) and some roasted cumin seeds 2 or 3 times a day.
- Take ½ gram powdered nutmeg twice along with buttermilk.

- A powder prepared from the dried flowers of the mango tree is recommended.
- The juice extracted from the juvenile leaves and flowers of *neem* is recommended.

FLU
Ayurvedic Name *Vatta Shlaishmika Jwara*

Characteristic Symptoms
- Fever with shivering, body aches and muscular pain, malaise and sore throat.
- Perhaps conjunctivitis and watering eyes.
- Perhaps inflammation of the bronchi, nose and larynx and gastro-intestinal disturbances.

Ayurvedic View
Vitiation in either of the three body humors that is particularly influenced by change of seasons and rainfall results in production of this disease. Other than this, factors like sensitivity of the throat, nasal mucous, tendency towards constipation and decrease in body resistance make the body more prone to the infection.

Management by Home Cures
- Mix 1 tsp raw turmeric powder in a glass of hot milk: Take twice a day.
- Mix fresh juice of ginger with 1 tsp honey and approx. 2 pinches of freshly ground black pepper and take 2 or 3 times.
- Boil a few basil leaves and ¼ tsp dried ginger powder to prepare a decoction. Take warm twice or thrice, with some *mishri* powder or honey added if preferred.
- Prepare a mixture of ½ tsp powdered long pepper, ½ tsp ginger juice and 1 tsp honey. Take every 4 to 8 hours in accordance with the severity of the symptoms.

SPRUCE
Ayurvedic Name *Sangrahani*

Characteristic Symptoms
- Loose stools, perhaps after intake of food.
- Perhaps pain in the abdomen, flatus, abdominal distention, nausea and feeling of incomplete evacuation.
- Stools with semi-digested or undigested wastes.
- Sore tongue, loss of appetite and weight loss in long-lasting ailment.
- Large quantity of stools passed generally in the mornings; flakes of mucous may be present in the stools.

Ayurvedic View
This disease is caused by vitiation of the fire or *pitta dosha*. Impairment of the functions of the inner wall of the intestine, wrong dietary habits and increased stress are other causes. The mixing up of the vitiated humors with the bowels make the intestines weak.

Management by Home Cures
- Before meals, slowly chew a spoonful of black sesame seeds and slowly swallow the juice.
- Take ½ to 1 g powdered nutmeg twice a day.
- Approx. 1 tsp of flea seed husk can be taken along with buttermilk.
- Increase the intake of buttermilk (fat removed), adding a pinch each of freshly ground black pepper, roasted cumin seeds and roasted coriander seeds.

- Take 1 to 2 tsp powdered *bilva* seeds twice or thrice.
- Take 50 ml of the fresh juice of radish and carrot mixed in equal quantities, twice.
- Roast a piece of dried ginger and some fennel in cow's ghee; pound together. Take 1 tsp of this mixture twice a day with some *mishri* powder added to it.
- Prepare a *halwa* (dessert) from the flour of *singhara* (water chestnut). Take twice daily for some days.

SORE TONGUE
Ayurvedic Name *Jihvapaka*

Characteristic Symptoms
- Inflammation of the mucous membrane of the tongue.
- Tongue becomes red and sore and ulcers may exist.
- Difficulty in eating food.

Ayurvedic View
This disease is caused by an aggravation in the fire body humor. Constipated bowels add to the predisposing cause.

Management by Home Cures
- Apply the milk of raw papaya on the tongue 2 to 3 times a day.
- Gargles and mouth-rinses with powdered *phitkari* mixed in water are recommended.
- Take approx. ½ tsp turmeric powder either with water or mixed in a glassful of milk once or twice.
- Local massage with powdered camphor twice daily is recommended.
- Pound a piece of camphor into a fine powder. Add some glycerine and use this mixture for local application on the tongue.
- Mash a ripe banana and add to a cup of curd (yogurt). Take this twice a day.
- Boil the bark of the pomegranate tree to prepare a decoction. Gargle with this 2 or 3 times a day.
- Drink rose water or gargle with it 2 or 3 times a day.

HAEMORRHAGE
Ayurvedic Name   *Rakta Pitta*

Characteristic Symptoms
- External or internal expulsion of blood due to injury or some disorder of an internal body organ.
- Shock in case of severe loss of vital fluid.
- Perhaps appearance of blood in vomiting or from other orifices.

Ayurvedic View
The disease of *Rakta Pitta* is believed to be a manifestation of the vitiation of the fire body humor in the blood, which further causes a distortion of the blood.

Management by Home Cures
- Take 20 to 30 ml of the freshly extracted juice of *amla* twice or thrice a day.
- Coconut water can be taken in unlimited quantities.
- Take approx. 50 ml of the juice of pomegranate 2 or 3 times a day.
- Take 20 to 30 ml of the juice of *petha* thrice a day.
- Pound *shankhpushpi* with some water to extract the juice or to make a paste: Take approx. 20 ml, twice.
- Sprinkle the powder of catechu at the site of bleeding to arrest the blood loss.
- Local application of powdered alum at the site of blood loss aids in ceasing the same.
- Take half teaspoon each of alum powder and turmeric powder mixed into a glass of hot milk once or twice a day.

THIRST

Ayurvedic Name   *Trishna Roga*

Characteristic Symptoms

- Feeling of unquenched thirst with increased need to drink water.
- Signs of dehydration in advanced cases.

Ayurvedic View

This disease is believed to emerge from vitiation of all the 3 humors.

1. When *vatta* is aggravated, there is a feeling of pain and giddiness along with acute thirst.
2. When *pitta* is aggravated, there is burning in the throat and chest.
3. When *kapha* is distorted, there is increased thirst, nausea and the presence of a salty taste in the mouth.

Management by Home Cures

- Take 20 ml fresh juice of *amla* twice a day.
- Take coconut water 3 or 4 times daily.
- Pound the seeds of large a cardamom to make a powder. Take 1 to 3 g along with warm water, twice.
- Heat a cleaned piece of brick on the fire and when hot, immerse it in water. Filter this water and take 2 or 3 times.
- A sweetened drink called *panna* prepared by boiling raw mangoes helps to quench thirst.

- Take the essence or syrup of sandalwood 2 or 3 times a day.
- Fresh juice of lemon can be sucked, or sweetened lime water can be taken 2 or 3 times to find relief.
- Take approx. 5 to 10 g of powdered seeds of *singhara* (water chestnut) 2 or 3 times with water.
- Add the juice of ripe tamarind to sugar and make a syrup. Cool and take 15 to 20 ml every 4 to 6 hours.
- Take 10 to 20 ml of the juice extracted from slightly raw *petha* twice a day.
- Basil leaves can be chewed. Or, boil them in water, allow to cool gradually, then add *mishri* and take 2 or 3 times.

DEFECTIVE EYESIGHT
Ayurvedic Name   *Drishti Dosha*

Characteristic Symptoms
- Difficulty in seeing, especially far-off objects.
- Perhaps blurred vision, particularly with regard to distant objects.
- Occasional headaches and loss of sleep in long-term cases.

Ayurvedic View
This vision problem is caused by nervous debility and also by prolonged constipation and a common cold.

Management by Home Cures
- Extract the juice from the fresh fruit of *amla*. Take 20 ml twice a day.
- Mix 1 tsp powdered asparagus in ½ tsp honey. Take twice daily along with warmed cow's milk.
- Local application of a paste or oil of *amla* or *bhringraj* on the scalp is good for the eyesight.
- Regular intake of powdered black pepper with some honey gives better vision.
- Pound some fresh coriander and apply the juice on the eyelids, repeating for several days to alleviate eye strain.
- Rub the soles of the feet with some oil or ghee regularly.
- The juice extracted from fresh garlic is used for regaining lost eyesight.

- Take mango regularly during the season as it is rich in vitamin A and will alleviate eye strain.
- Fresh juice extracted from properly cleaned rose petals is believed to improve the vision. This can be used both externally and internally.
- Wash your eyes regularly with a decoction of *trifla* powder.
- Take approx. ½ to 1 tsp powdered liquorice twice daily along with cow's milk. It can also to be taken mixed with honey or ghee.

CONJUNCTIVITIS
Ayurvedic Name *Netra Abhishyanda*

Characteristic Symptoms
- Inflammation of the conjunctivae along with discomfort, grittiness and sticky eyelids.
- Purulent or watery discharge from the eyes.
- Intense itching and mucoid discharge if the problem is allergic.
- The ailment becomes chronic with regular exposure to dust, smoke and cold winds.

Ayurvedic View
This disease is caused by vitiation in the *vatta, pitta* and *kapha doshas* of the body. Sometimes conjunctivitis may result from vitiation in the blood or *rakta dhatu* when it is called *rakta abhishyanda*.

Management by Home Cures
- Take 3 to 6 g of the powder of the 3 myrobalans (*amla, harad* and *baheda*) twice a day.
- Use plain rose water on the eyelids or as eye drops.
- According to Ayurvedic texts, *bilva* leaves are beneficial in treating conjunctivitis. The fresh, clean juice extracted from the leaves of *bilva* should be properly filtered through a muslin cloth. Use as eye drops, or make a paste out of pounded leaves and apply to the eyelids.

- Prepare a decoction by boiling freshly dried coriander. Filter and use as an eye wash to treat the burning, oozing and redness of the eyes.
- Mix powdered alum into *gulab jala* (rose water); carefully filter it through a muslin cloth. Put 2 to 3 drops of this liquid into the eyes.
- Soak powder of the 3 myrobalans overnight. In the morning strain through a clean cloth. Use this liquid both for drinking and as an eye-wash; it helps most eye problems.

GREYING OF HAIR
Ayurvedic Name *Palitya*

Characteristic Symptoms
- Greying of the hair begins at a younger age.
- Premature greying portrays the person as much older than his actual age.

Ayurvedic View
This malady is caused by aggravation of the *pitta dosha* of the body. Factors like excessive anxiety, stress and anger are additional causes. Long-lasting gastric upsets as well as chronic cold and sinusitis are also some of the predisposing factors.

Management by Home Cures
- Daily massage of the scalp with the fingertips improves the blood circulation, strengthens the hair roots and also helps to delay discolouration of the hair.
- Take approx. 1 tsp of the powder of dried *amla* with honey twice a day. Wash the hair with *amla* powder.
- Add henna leaves to some mustard oil and heat gently to make an easy, homemade medicated hair oil.
- Mix powdered dried *amlas* in lemon juice, apply into the hair and massage on the scalp.
- A massage of sesame oil on the scalp improves hair growth and could prevent premature greying and hair loss.

- Pound dried *amlas* to make a powder and mix with water to make a paste. Apply this paste onto the hair half an hour before a head wash. Repeat 2 or 3 times a week.
- Mix approx. 100 g each of dried, powdered *amla*, *bhringraj*, *bramhi*, henna and *shikakai* into 1 kg coconut oil. Heat on a very low flame preferably in an iron pan till the mixture becomes smooth. Filter and use as hair oil everyday or on alternate days.
- Take 1 tsp of the powdered mixture of *amla*, *harad* and *baheda* preferably with lukewarm water once or twice daily for some days.